Obs and Gynae

PG Focus Series

Cardiac Diseases in Pregnancy

Obs and Gynae

PG Focus Series

Cardiac Diseases in Pregnancy

Editors

Niranjan Chavan

MD FICOG FCPS DGO DFP MICOG DICOG Diploma in Endoscopy (USA)

Professor and Unit Chief

Department of Obstetrics and Gynaecology

Lokmanya Tilak Medical College and General Hospital

Mumbai, Maharashtra, India

Komal N Chavan

MD DNB MNAMS FCPS DGO FICOG and Diploma in Reproductive Medicine (UK-SH Germany)

Senior Consultant and Unit Chief

Department of Obstetrics and Gynaecology

VN Desai Hospital

Mumbai, Maharashtra, India

Co-Editors

Tulika Chouhan

MBBS MS (Obs/Gynae) DNB MRCOG PDCC in Gynaecological Endoscopy

Senior Clinical Fellow

Department of Obstetrics and Gynaecology

Norfolk and Norwich University Hospital

England, UK

Sonam Simpatwar

MBBS MS (Obs/Gynae) DNB

DGO Advanced Diploma in ART and Reproductive Medicine, Kiel, Germany

Clinical Assistant

Department of Obstetrics and Gynaecology

Bharatratna Dr Babasaheb Ambedkar Municipal General Hospital

Mumbai, Maharashtra, India

JAYPEE

JAYPEE BROTHERS MEDICAL PUBLISHERS

The Health Sciences Publisher

New Delhi | London

Jaypee Brothers Medical Publishers (P) Ltd

Headquarters
Jaypee Brothers Medical Publishers (P) Ltd
EMCA House, 23/23-B
Ansari Road, Daryaganj
New Delhi 110 002, India
Landline: +91-11-23272143, +91-11-23272703
+91-11-23282021, +91-11-23245672
Email: jaypee@jaypeebrothers.com

Corporate Office
Jaypee Brothers Medical Publishers (P) Ltd
4838/24, Ansari Road, Daryaganj
New Delhi 110 002, India
Phone: +91-11-43574357
Fax: +91-11-43574314
Email: jaypee@jaypeebrothers.com

Overseas Office
JP Medical Ltd.
83, Victoria Street, London
SW1H 0HW (UK)
Phone: +44 20 3170 8910
Fax: +44 (0)20 3008 6180
Email: info@jpmedpub.com

Website: www.jaypeebrothers.com
Website: www.jaypeedigital.com

Inquiries for bulk sales may be solicited at: jaypee@jaypeebrothers.com

Obs and Gynae PG Focus Series: Cardiac Diseases in Pregnancy

First Edition: **2025**

ISBN: 978-93-6616-014-6

Printed in India

Preface

Medical residency is an intensive period of training where newly graduated doctors gain practical experience in their chosen specialties under the guidance of experienced physicians. This also is a challenging time, where young minds have to strike a balance between patient care, improving their clinical acumen as well as learning the theoretical aspects of their subject.

Heart disease during pregnancy presents unique challenges, as it requires managing both maternal and fetal health in the context of significant physiological change. Our goal is to bridge gaps in specialized care, ensuring that clinicians have access to comprehensive resources to help them navigate these complex cases with confidence and precision.

The increasing prevalence of cardiovascular conditions among women of childbearing age has made it imperative for clinicians to be equipped with the most current and evidence-based referral options.

Within this book, you will find resources organized by category and specialty, from preconception counseling to postpartum monitoring. This book encompasses up-to-date knowledge with clinically relevant data.

It is our hope that this book will serve as an invaluable asset, facilitating seamless collaboration among healthcare providers and enhancing the quality-of-care for mothers facing the dual journey of heart disease and pregnancy. We extend our deepest gratitude to the contributors and specialists whose work inspires and informs this book.

Editors
Niranjan Chavan
Komal N Chavan

Co-Editors
Tulika Chouhan
Sonam Simpatwar

Acknowledgments

We express our gratitude to all those who contributed to the completion of this book on Cardiac Diseases in Pregnancy. This endeavor would not have been possible without the constant support of many individuals.

We are thankful to all the authors and co-authors for sharing their expertise and commitment to producing a resource of the highest standards.

We are grateful to our mentors and colleagues, whose valuable guidance helped us form the structure and contents of this book.

Our deepest gratitude to our families and friends for their unwavering support, patience, and encouragement during the demanding phases of this project have been our greatest strength.

We acknowledge the support of Shri Jitendar P Vij (Group Chairman) and Mr Ankit Vij (Managing Director) of M/s Jaypee Brothers Medical Publishers (P) Ltd, New Delhi, India, in publishing the book and their associates, particularly Ms Chetna Malhotra (Senior Director—Professional Publishing, Marketing, and Business Development), Ms Kritika Dua (Senior Commissioning Editor), and Ms Pragati Singh (Development Editor), who have been prompt, efficient, and most helpful.

Lastly, we hope that the postgraduate students find this book useful in their examinations and teachers for a quick revision. We also hope this book serves as a valuable resource, contributing to the betterment of patient care and surgical practice to the practicing obstetricians and gynaecologists.

Thank you all for being a part of this journey.

Contents

1 CHAPTER

Cardiovascular Physiology of Pregnancy

INTRODUCTION

Pregnancy is a dynamic process associated with significant physiological changes in the cardiovascular system. The increased metabolic demands of the mother and fetus are met through these changes by ensuring adequate uteroplacental circulation for fetal growth and development. Preeclampsia and intrauterine growth retardation result if the hemodynamic changes are insufficient.

Pregnancy is associated with vasodilation of the systemic and renal vasculature. Peripheral vascular resistance reduces significantly in the first trimester, reaches a low in the middle of the second trimester, and then plateaus or slightly increases for the duration of the pregnancy. The reduction is between 35 and 40% of the baseline. Systemic vascular resistance returns to prepregnancy levels 2 weeks after birth. Increased vascular compliance has been observed in normal human pregnancy starting in the first trimester. In the postpartum period, the systemic vascular resistance increases to the normal prepregnancy level. By the end of the first trimester there is a decrease in serum creatinine, urea, and uric acid values as renal blood flow and glomerular filtration rate is increased due to vasodilatation.[1]

Cardiovascular changes have been discussed under following subheading.

CARDIAC OUTPUT

There is increase in cardiac output throughout pregnancy. To measure cardiac output mother is generally made to lie in left lateral decubitus position to avoid variation due to position.

By the beginning of the first trimester, there is a significant increase in cardiac output, which continues until the second trimester. In a typical, singleton pregnancy, the increase in cardiac output can be up to 45% by 24 weeks.

When compared to singleton pregnancy, twin pregnancy results in a 15% increase in cardiac output, resulting in an increase in left atrial diameter, which is consistent with volume overload. Early in pregnancy, an increase in stroke volume is mediated by an increase in heart rate, while later in pregnancy is mediated by an increase in cardiac output. The stroke volume increases gradually during pregnancy until the end of the second trimester,

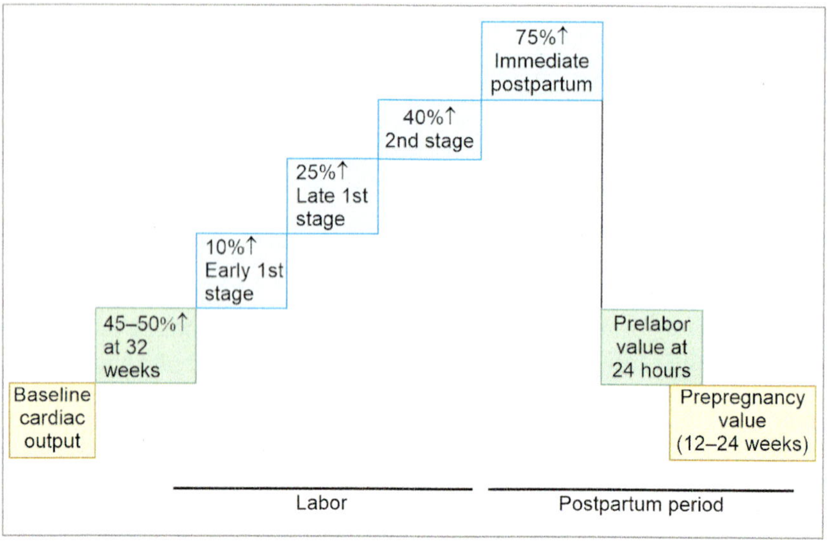

Fig. 1: Increase in cardiac output during pregnancy, labor, and postpartum period.
Source: Bhatia P, Chhabra S. Physiological and anatomical changes of pregnancy: Implications for anaesthesia. Indian J Anaesthesia. 2018;62(9):651-7.

after which it remains steady or declines late in the pregnancy. **Figure 1** shows the trend in increase in cardiac output during pregnancy, labor, and postpartum period.

BLOOD PRESSURE

Systolic blood pressure, diastolic blood pressure, and mean arterial pressure decreases during pregnancy. The fall in diastolic and mean arterial pressure is more than the fall in systolic blood pressure. Maximum fall in arterial pressure occurs in second trimester.

HEART RATE

During normal pregnancy, the heart rate rises by 10–20 beats per minute, peaking in the third trimester. The overall rise in heart rate is between 20 and 25% over baseline.

CONTRACTILITY

Although multiple cardiovascular parameters are altered during pregnancy, myocardial contractility, and ejection fractions do not appear to change during pregnancy.

SYMPATHETIC ACTIVITY AND BARORECEPTORS

Vasomotor sympathetic activity is increases, and this increase occurs very early in pregnancy. Normal pregnancy appears to be associated with increased maternal baroreceptor sensitivity and an attenuated responsiveness to α-adrenergic stimulation.

PREGNANCY HORMONAL CHANGES

Hormones (estrogen and progesterone) have been demonstrated to have an endothelium-dependent vasodilatory role in pregnancy that can influence small arterial resistance vessels. Although nitric oxide plays a crucial part in the reproductive system's physiology, its role in mediating the systemic vasodilation seen during human pregnancy is unknown.[2]

RENIN–ANGIOTENSIN–ALDOSTERONE SYSTEM

The renin-angiotensin-aldosterone system is activated throughout a normal pregnancy. The renin-angiotensin-aldosterone system is more active, with increases in plasma volume beginning at 6–8 weeks and continuing until 28–30 weeks. During pregnancy, the generation of renin substrate (angiotensinogen) rises, resulting in an increase in angiotensin levels. This helps retain salt and water in pregnancy, which maintains blood pressure, as maternal systemic and renal arterial dilation (with resulting salt and water loss) creates an "underfilled" cardiovascular system. Furthermore, during pregnancy, relaxin stimulates increased vasopressin secretion and drinking, resulting in increased water retention. There is hyponatremic hypervolemia in pregnancy in spite of increase in exchangeable sodium. Progesterone acts on the mineralocorticoid receptor as a potent aldosterone antagonist and helps in preventing sodium retention and to protects against hypokalemia. Maternal plasma atrial natriuretic peptide levels increases in the third trimester, suggesting a significant role in postpartum diuresis.[3]

CHANGES IN PLASMA VOLUME AND RED BLOOD CELL MASS

Total blood volume, plasma volume, and red cell mass increases during pregnancy to provide nutrition. Erythropoiesis maybe enhanced by effect of placental lactogen. This increase is more when red cell, hemoglobin is lower and subclinical iron deficiency exists. The decreased life span of red blood cells also results in increased production.

Reduced plasma volume expansion has been linked to preeclampsia and other pathological diseases, and there is a clear link between plasma volume expansion and fetal growth. Blood volume rises dramatically in the first few weeks of pregnancy and continues to rise steadily throughout the pregnancy. The overall blood volume increase ranges from 20 to 100% above prepregnancy levels, with the average being about 45%. There is a 40% increase in red blood cell synthesis via erythropoiesis. Physiological anemia occurs when the volume of plasma expands higher than the volume of red blood cells, resulting in physiological dilution.

REMODELING

Left ventricular wall thickness and left ventricular wall mass increase throughout pregnancy. Increased vascular distensibility, aortic augmentation index, a marker of aortic stiffness, decreases significantly early during pregnancy, due to systemic vasodilation, reaching a nadir in the second trimester and gradually increasing in the third trimester.

TRANSTHORACIC ECHOCARDIOGRAPHY AND CARDIOVASCULAR MAGNETIC RESONANCE

Mild four-chamber dilatation (changes in the right atrium and ventricle are often higher than those in the left atrium and ventricle) is common during pregnancy, along with trivial mitral regurgitation and physiological tricuspid and pulmonary regurgitation. The most common imaging technique used in pregnancy is echocardiography, which is safe in all three trimesters.

A cardiac MRI is a better indication of left ventricular volume. When compared to cardiovascular magnetic resonance, echocardiography underestimates left ventricular mass, cardiac output, and stroke volume.

Finally, in pregnant patients with suspected cardiovascular problems, cardiovascular magnetic resonance of the atria, right ventricle, and aorta is probably more accurate than echocardiography and should be explored on a case-by-case basis.[4]

LABOR AND DELIVERY

Many factors contribute to the greatest increase in cardiac output during labor and immediately after delivery, including an increase in heart rate and preload caused by uterine contraction pain, increased circulating catecholamine, and auto transfusion of 300–500 mL of blood from the uterus into systemic circulation.

Spinal anesthesia can have serious side effects on the heart and blood vessels. A considerable drop in systemic vascular resistance and compensatory increases in heart rate and stroke volume are the most common responses to spinal anesthesia during caesarean section. In obstetrics, phenylephrine is preferred over ephedrine as a vasopressor.

CLINICAL CARDIOVASCULAR FINDINGS IN NORMAL PREGNANCY

Shortness of breath and increased fatigue can be experienced by normal woman during pregnancy. As resting cardiac output is increased in pregnancy, maximal cardiac output induced by exercise is achieved at lower level of work. During rest or weight bearing exercise, there is significant increase in maternal oxygen consumption.

In the respiratory system, the tidal volume and resting minute ventilation are increased and expiratory reserve volume and functional residual capacity is reduced.

TABLE 1: Changes in electrocardiogram and cardiac auscultation during pregnancy.[5]

Changes in cardiac auscultation	*Changes in electrocardiogram*
• Loud S_1 • Ejection systolic murmur • S_3 and S_4 (no clinical significance)	• Shortened PR and QT interval • Shifted QRS axis • Rightward (first trimester) • Leftward (third trimester) • ST segment depression • Isoelectric low-voltage T waves in both precordial and limb leads

Source: Bhatia P, Chhabra S. Physiological and anatomical changes of pregnancy: Implications for anaesthesia. Indian J Anaesthesia. 2018;62(9):651-7.

Physiological anemia of pregnancy develops as a result of increase in plasma volume more than that of red blood cell mass with increased vasopressin secretion causing water retention leading to hyponatremic hypervolemic state of pregnancy. As a result, gestation-dependent edema can be found in up to 80% of healthy pregnant women.

In 90% of cases, an ejection systolic flow murmur is heard, a third heart sound is heard in 80% of cases, and an atrioventricular diastolic flow murmur is heard in 20% of cases.

In a normal pregnancy, electrocardiogram (ECG) changes include an increase in resting heart rate and a little shift in the QRS complex (left or right). **Table 1** highlights the ECG changes in pregnancy.

CONCLUSION

The cardiovascular system undergoes significant structural and hemodynamic changes which are necessary for fetal growth and development, failure to achieve which can lead to fetal and maternal morbidity.

REFERENCES

1. Mahendru AA, Everett TR, Wilkinson IB, Lees CC, McEniery CM. A longitudinal study of maternal cardiovascular function from preconception to the postpartum period. J Hypertens. 2014;32:849-56.
2. Chapman AB, Abraham WT, Zamudio S, Coffin C, Merouani A, Young D, et al. Temporal relationships between hormonal and hemodynamic changes in early human pregnancy. Kidney Int. 1998;54:2056-63.
3. Baker PN, Broughton Pipkin F, Symonds EM. Platelet angiotensin II binding and plasma renin concentration, plasma renin substrate and plasma angiotensin II in human pregnancy. Clin Sci (Lond). 1990;79:403-8.
4. Bellenger NG, Burgess MI, Ray SG, Lahiri A, Coats AJ, Cleland JG, et al. Comparison of left ventricular ejection fraction and volumes in heart failure by echocardiography, radionuclide ventriculography and cardiovascular magnetic resonance; are they interchangeable? Eur Heart J. 2000;21:1387-96.
5. Bhatia P, Chhabra S. Physiological and anatomical changes of pregnancy: Implications for anaesthesia. Indian J Anaesthesia. 2018;62(9):651-7.

CHAPTER 2

Prepregnancy Counseling

INTRODUCTION

Prepregnancy counseling aims to inform women about the risks that pregnancy may pose to their health and that of their fetus, such as deterioration of functional class during pregnancy, risk of thromboembolism, arrhythmia, heart failure, negative impact on the fetus, and the need for medication changes.

It allows any risk-reducing or prognostically meaningful action to be performed prior to conception.

It is appropriate for some women to talk about the risk of inheritance.

PREPREGNANCY ASSESSMENT

Access to previous notes, particularly any previous operation notes, is vital when evaluating any woman to estimate the risk of a future pregnancy. A complete physical examination and functional assessment should be performed:

- Classification by functionality [New York Heart Association (NYHA) classes I and II generally predict a good outcome]
- Resting oxygen saturations
- X-ray of the chest
- An electrocardiogram (ECG)
- Echocardiography
- Oxygen saturation monitoring during exercise
- Evaluation of B-type natriuretic protein (BNP) and pro-BNP
- As needed, cardiac magnetic resonance imaging (CMRI)/angiography

MEDICATION

To lessen the risk of a neural tube abnormality, women should be taught about the importance of starting folic acid before to conception (current recommended 400 mg when trying to conceive until 3 months of pregnancy). Angiotensin-converting enzyme (ACE) inhibitors as well as warfarin, statins, and spironolactone are all teratogenic medicines that should be avoided before conception.

FETAL RISK

Cardiac disease in the mother is associated with risk of preterm delivery and fetal growth restriction. Predictors of adverse outcome are maternal

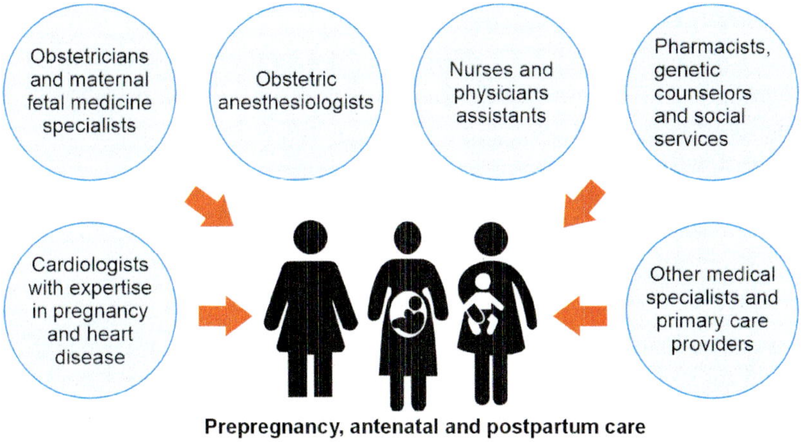

Fig. 1: Multidisciplinary team involvement in care.[2]
Source: Sharma G, Ying W, Silversides CK. The Importance of Cardiovascular Risk Assessment and Pregnancy Heart Team in the Management of Cardiovascular Disease in Pregnancy. Cardiol Clin. 2021;39(1):7-19.

cyanosis, oral anticoagulants, left heart obstruction, maternal smoking, and mechanical heart valve replacement.[1]

Other than the earlier mentioned, fetus is also at risk of exposure to teratogenic medications. Fetus is at risk of congenital heart disease if the same has been diagnosed in the mother without chromosomal abnormalities.

Figure 1 shows the involvement of multidisciplinary team for care of woman with heart disease, beginning from preconceptional care, antenatal care, and postpartum care.

INDIVIDUAL CARDIAC CONDITIONS

Ischemic Heart Disease

There is three- to fourfold increased risk and the majority is anterior infarcts. Prior to pregnancy it is necessary to revascularize patients with inducible ischemia. If there is a left ventricular impairment as a result of ischemia the risk stratification should be according to the degree of impairment.

Turner Syndrome

With a poor maternal and fetal outcome, there is a higher chance of cardiovascular issues later in life. Prior to oocyte donation, the American Society for Reproductive Medicine recommends that women with Turner syndrome undergo cardiovascular screening. A 24-hour blood pressure reading, a transthoracic echo, and a whole-aorta MRI should all be part of the patient's examination. The management of a pregnancy with Turner syndrome necessitates a multidisciplinary approach.[3]

Peripartum Cardiomyopathy

It is a nonfamilial and nongenetic cardiomyopathy associated with pregnancy. The outcome from peripartum cardiomyopathy (PPCM) is superior when at diagnosis:

- Ejection fraction >30%
- End-diastolic dimension of the left ventricle is 5.5 cm
- The cardiac troponin level is particularly low
- A troponin level measured 2 weeks after a diagnosis was found to be related to the ejection fraction 6 months later

Recurrence is the most significant danger; hence all patients with PPCM should get prepregnancy counseling. When a woman has:

- Poor systolic function (ejection fraction 25%) at the time of diagnosis, she should be advised against having another child.
- At 6 months after diagnosis, left ventricular function has not recovered. Patient should be made aware of risk of deterioration of left ventricular function in further pregnancy which might not recover.[4]

OBSTRUCTIVE LEFT HEART CONDITIONS

Aortic Stenosis

Women with mild aortic stenosis are low risk. Women with severe aortic stenosis should be informed that pregnancy is contraindicated and moderate to severe stenosis require proper assessment. Women with moderate or severe aortic stenosis who have had a pregnancy should be counseled about the higher risk of late cardiac events compared to nonpregnant women during prepregnancy counseling.[5]

Mitral Stenosis

Moderate or severe mitral stenosis is poorly tolerated as there is already volume overloading and tachycardia in pregnancy. This is associated with significant morbidity. Pregnancy should be delayed until the valve is intervened on, ideally with balloon valvuloplasty where appropriate.

Mitral and Aortic Regurgitation

Regurgitant lesions are well tolerated in pregnancy due to a decrease in systemic vascular resistance, as long as the mother has good left ventricular function, appropriate pulmonary pressures, and a normal exercise capacity.

Prosthetic Valve Replacements

Despite the fact that a bioprosthesis does not require formal anticoagulation, it has a short valve lifespan in younger patients and is linked to structural degradation. All women of reproductive age who require valve surgery should get expert advice on the sort of valve replacement that is best for them.[6]

Warfarin is the best protection against maternal thrombosis, which can be fatal to both the mother and the fetus if not taken during pregnancy. Warfarin is also linked to a significant increase in the risk of fetal loss, deformity, and preterm delivery.

Heparin does not cross the placenta, although it is linked to an increased risk of maternal valve thrombosis and thromboembolism, as well as osteoporosis and thrombocytopenia in the mother. Unfractionated heparin regimens caused more thromboembolism, thus they have been replaced by twice-daily, weight-adjusted, and low molecular weight heparin (LMWH) regimens with routine anti-Xa level monitoring. For metallic valve replacements, there is no single acknowledged anticoagulation strategy, and a customized plan should take into account the patient's wishes and medical history.

Congenital Heart Disease

Those with experience in congenital cardiac disease should provide prepregnancy counseling. In general, pregnant women who saturate well, are in a good functional class, and have normal left ventricular function perform well.

Pulmonary Hypertension

Pulmonary hypertension (PHT), defined as a mean pulmonary pressure of 25 mm Hg at rest or 30 mm Hg during exercise as measured by a cardiac catheter, is a difficult and progressing condition. While this is a step forward, mortality is still a possibility, and several targeted therapy medications, such as bosentan and ambrisentan, are teratogens. In a PHT center, careful counseling is required.

CONCLUSION

Prepregnancy counseling should be seen as the cornerstone of therapeutic management, and it should begin early in the transition period for women with congenital heart disease. Despite the fact that women with cardiac disease are at higher risk during pregnancy, the majority of women enjoy a healthy pregnancy.

If a woman is advised to avoid or terminate a pregnancy, she should be reassured that she will continue to be supported and cared for if she chooses to carry the pregnancy to term.

REFERENCES

1. Gelson E, Curry R, Gatzoulis MA, Swan L, Lupton M, Steer P, et al. Effect of maternal heart disease on fetal growth. Obstet Gynecol. 2011;117:886-91.

2. Sharma G, Ying W, Silversides CK. The Importance of Cardiovascular Risk Assessment and Pregnancy Heart Team in the Management of Cardiovascular Disease in Pregnancy. Cardiol Clin. 2021;39(1):7-19.
3. Chevalier N, Ltur H, Lelannou D, Ohl J, Cornet D, Chalas-Boissonnas C, et al. Materno-fetal cardiovascular complications in Turner syndrome after oocyte donation: insufficient prepregnancy screening and pregnancy follow-up are associated with poor outcome. J Clin Endocrinol Metab. 2011;96: E260-7.
4. Van Spaendonck-Zwarts KY, van Tintelen JP, van Veldhuisen DJ, van der Werf R, Jongbloed JD, Paulus WJ, et al. Peripartum cardiomyopathy as a part of familial dilated cardiomyopathy. Circulation. 2010;121:2169-75.
5. Silversides C, Colman J, Sermer M, Farine D, Siu SC. Early and intermediate-term outcomes of pregnancy with congenital aortic stenosis. Am J Cardiol. 2003;91:1386-9.
6. McLintock C, McCowan LME, North RA. Maternal complications and pregnancy outcome in women with mechanical prosthetic heart valves treated with enoxaparin. BJOG. 2009;116(12):1585-92.

CHAPTER 3

Valvular Heart Disease

CASE SCENARIO

A 38-year-old pregnant woman was admitted with a severe cough and exacerbated dyspnea in the 37th week of her pregnancy. At the age of 31 years, she was diagnosed with rheumatic heart disease (RHD). She presented with RHD, significant mitral stenosis, secondary pulmonary hypertension, and heart failure at 37 weeks of pregnancy. As a result, the patient had an emergency caesarean delivery followed by a reoperative mitral valve replacement, which was completed successfully while the patient was on cardiopulmonary bypass (CPB).[1]

INTRODUCTION

Valvular heart disease is commonly seen complicating pregnancy and is an important cause of maternal mortality.

In developing countries, it is most commonly seen as a consequence of childhood rheumatic fever.[2]

It may be diagnosed earlier or present first during pregnancy.

- Stenotic lesions are not well tolerated during pregnancy and labor as there is limitation to the ability of heart to increase cardiac output.
- Regurgitant lesions are generally better tolerated.

Table 1 summarizes various valvular lesions and their symptoms.

STENOTIC LESIONS

The most commonly affected valve following acute rheumatic fever is the mitral valve.

- The leading cause of maternal mortality in developing countries is mitral stenosis as it is poorly tolerated during pregnancy.
- Due to physiological changes of pregnancy, symptoms are precipitated, usually in mid second trimester.
- Symptoms include dyspnea on exertion and postural symptoms such as orthopnea and paroxysmal nocturnal dyspnea. Classical features of mid diastolic murmur at apex may be difficult to diagnose during pregnancy due to pulmonary edema or rapid tachycardia.
- Investigations include radiological signs of an enlarged left atrium and electrocardiogram (ECG) evidence of a bifid P wave, pregnancy results

TABLE 1: Types of valvular disorders and symptoms.[6]

Valvular disorder	*Description*	*Stage D symptoms*
Aortic stenosis	Narrowed aortic valvular disorder that results in reduced blood flow through the valve	Exertional dyspnea, angina, syncope, and heart failure (HF)
Aortic regurgitation	Valvular disorder that allows blood flow back into the left ventricle	Exertional dyspnea or angina or more severe HF symptoms
Mitral stenosis	Narrowed mitral valvular disorder that results in reduced blood flow through the valve	Decreased exercise tolerance and exertional dyspnea
Acute mitral regurgitation	Acute valvular disorder that allows blood flow back into the left atrium and pulmonary veins during systole	Decreased exercise tolerance and exertional dyspnea
Chronic mitral regurgitation	Gradual valvular disorder that allows blood flow back into the left atrium and pulmonary veins during systole	Decreased exercise tolerance, exertional dyspnea, HF symptoms due to mitral regurgitation persist even after revascularization, and therapy optimization
Tricuspid regurgitation	Valvular disorder that allows blood flow back into the right atrium during systole	Fatigue, palpitations, dyspnea, abdominal bloating, anorexia, and edema

Source: Otto CM, Nishimura RA, Bonow RO, Carabello BA, Erwin JP 3rd, Gentile F, et al. 2020 AHA/ACC guideline for the management of patients with valvular heart disease: executive summary: a report of the American College of Cardiology/American Heart Association Joint Committee on Clinical Practice Guidelines. Circulation. 2021;2021;143(5):e35-71.

in a mitralized cardiac shadow in the absence of any valvular pathology making diagnosis difficult.

- Due to pregnancy-related tachycardia and the increased blood volume, degree of mitral stenosis can be increased, resulting in increase in pulmonary capillary pressures.
- Increases in systemic vascular resistance of the third trimester which increases left-sided filling pressures further increases chances of pulmonary edema.
- Due to left atrial dilatation the risk of atrial fibrillation increases. Because of an increasingly hyperdynamic circulation and the acute increase in blood volume during the third stage of labor, the risk of pulmonary edema increases even more during labor and immediately after delivery.
- Patients with left atrial dilatation are also at an increased risk of developing intracardiac thrombus, and should be anticoagulated with therapeutic low-molecular-weight heparin (LMWH).[3]

MANAGEMENT

Controlling the heart rate, restricting volume expansion, and preventing the development of comorbidity owing to anemia, hyperthyroidism, and sepsis are all principles of medical care. Beta-blockade prevents arrhythmias and prolongs diastolic filling of the left ventricle, in addition to regulating heart rate.

Prompt rate control is required in atrial fibrillation and atrial flutter, and early cardio version should be considered. Reflex tachycardia can develop due to afterload reduction further decreasing the diastolic filling time.

There is a risk of declining cardiac output with preload reduction. Patients with severe mitral stenosis are the ones who are more likely to decompensate (valve area $<1.0\ cm^2$).

In these patients and those who remain symptomatic despite medical treatment:

- *Elective percutaneous balloon valvuloplasty:* For patients where valve is suitable for the procedure, it should be considered in second trimester, before 20 weeks of gestation.
- Patients with moderate stenosis (valve area $1.0–1.5\ cm^2$) require close monitoring as they may require intervention. Mitral regurgitation, which develops during valvotomy, is usually better tolerated than a stenotic disease.
  - Echocardiographic finding which are significant are the mobility, thickness, and degree of calcification of the valvular structure. Calcification of the commissures (Wilkies score) or significant mitral regurgitation makes the valve unsuitable for valvuloplasty.
  - Closed commissurotomy is an alternative to percutaneous valvuloplasty when percutaneous valvuloplasty is not an option. Open-heart surgery is only performed when there are no other options and the mother's life is in danger.

Aortic stenosis (AS) this is an uncommon disorder with a poor prognosis when diagnosed during pregnancy. It is most usually related with congenital bicuspid aortic valve (which may be linked to aortopathy and the risk of aortic dissection) and is not caused by rheumatic disease.

Prepregnancy counseling plays an important role in patient where it is diagnosed before conception allowing counseling, optimization before pregnancy, and planning antenatal management.

Echocardiography is used for estimating severity of AS, quantification of AS and measurement of aortic diameter, is to be performed before pregnancy.

Exercise testing is recommended for asymptomatic patients to evaluate exercise tolerance, blood pressure response, arrhythmias, and need for intervention.

Absence of symptoms, normal ECG, normal exertional blood pressure rise, aortic valve area ≥1 cm^2, and normal left ventricular function, all are predictors of favorable outcome of pregnancy.

Pregnancy is usually well tolerated in asymptomatic AS, even if the condition is severe, as long as the patient stays asymptomatic throughout exercise tests and has a normal blood pressure response.

When left ventricular size and function, as well as the exercise test result, are normal, pregnancy should not be avoided in asymptomatic patients, even in severe AS. Breathlessness, syncope, chest pain, deterioration in left ventricular ejection fraction, a reduction or failure to increase transvalvular gradient (which should typically grow by 20% during pregnancy), and/or ischemic ECG abnormalities can all be signs of cardiac disease.

Valvuloplasty or corrective surgery needs to be performed in symptomatic patients with severe AS or asymptomatic patients with impaired left ventricular function or a pathological exercise test.[4]

To avoid presyncope, syncope, and hypotension, diuretics and cautious beta-blockade should be begun at a modest initial dose. Vasodilators should be avoided if at all possible. If medical therapy fails, birth of the fetus should be considered if gestational age permits, as this results in a significant improvement in the maternal cardiac state.

With severe symptoms and noncalcified valve, a percutaneous valvuloplasty can be undertaken.

For life-threatening symptoms, a valve replacement should be done after early delivery by caesarean procedure, if this is an option.

For severe symptomatic cases, delivery by caesarean delivery should be considered.

REGURGITANT LESIONS

Due to peripheral vasodilatation in pregnancy, the effect of mitral regurgitation is usually ameliorated in early pregnancy. There is increased plasma volume with reduction in systemic vascular resistance and consequently, the extent of the regurgitation diminishes.

In the middle of the third trimester, a rise in peripheral vascular resistance combined with a peak in plasma volume may cause increasing regurgitation and the start of symptoms and signs associated with fluid overload or pulmonary edema. Similar cardiovascular symptoms may be triggered by hypertension at an earlier stage of plasma volume expansion.

These patients normally respond well to diuretic medication and do not require any additional treatment to ensure the pregnancy's success. Patients with severe regurgitation should be evaluated to determine the risks and advantages of surgery, as well as the timing of the procedure in relation to pregnancy. Patients with left ventricular systolic dysfunction or pulmonary hypertension are at a higher risk of maternal and fetal problems. An enlarged left atrium raises the risk of atrial fibrillation. Valve repair should be offered to women of reproductive age with severe mitral regurgitation whenever possible, to minimize the hazards of bioprosthetic valve degeneration and early repeat surgery, as well as anticoagulation, thrombosis, and embolism associated with mechanical valves. A woman who is symptomatic and is not a candidate for valve repair or replacement should not become pregnant.

AORTIC REGURGITATION

This is less common, and those with rheumatic etiology often have mitral involvement as well. Bicuspid aortic valve is also the most common cause of aortic regurgitation (AR) in women of reproductive age. The symptoms and treatment are identical to mitral regurgitation during pregnancy. Chronic, moderate, or even severe AR is usually adequately tolerated if left ventricular function is retained. During pregnancy, women with severe AR are at risk for pulmonary edema and arrhythmias. Valve replacement during pregnancy is uncommon and should only be considered in symptomatic women who have failed to respond to conventional treatment.[5]

The management of mixed valvular lesion depends on dominant abnormality. Stenotic lesions are more likely to develop complications when compared to regurgitant lesions and left-sided cardiac valvular disease is associated with greater risk.

Prosthetic valves and bioprosthetic valves when compared to mechanical valves, which are linked to major maternal and fetal problems, provide negligible risks during pregnancy. Thrombosis and sepsis are two hazards associated with mechanical prosthetic valves. The prothrombotic profile of pregnancy raises the risk of thrombotic events, and the conflicting goal is to maintain anticoagulation while preserving the fetus from anticoagulant drug exposure and avoiding excessive bleeding during delivery.[7]

Table 2 highlights the differences between mechanical and bioprosthetic valve.

TABLE 2: Differences between mechanical valve versus bioprosthetic valve.[8]

	Mechanical valves	*Bioprosthetic valves*
Types	*Tilting-disc bileaflet*	*Heterografts (porcine or bovine)*
Durability	20–30 years	10–15 years
Subsequent valve replacement or repair	Lower risk	Higher risk
Thromboembolism	Higher risk	Lower risk
Anticoagulation	Lifelong	Minimum 3 months

Source: Tillquist MN, Maddox TM. Cardiac crossroads: deciding between mechanical or bioprosthetic heart valve replacement. Patient Prefer Adherence. 2011;5:91-9.

When administered early in pregnancy, warfarin crosses the placenta, causing embryopathy, fetal anticoagulation, and an increased risk of pregnancy loss in all three trimesters. Because heparin does not cross the placenta, it protects the unborn by anticoagulating only the mother; nevertheless, unfractionated heparin can only be used as an intravenous infusion, and the use of LMWH necessitates anti-Xa activity monitoring to ensure that the patient is in the therapeutic range. Warfarin is the most effective drug for preventing maternal valve thrombosis, but it also comes with the highest risk of miscarriage. There is a risk of osteoporosis and heparin-induced thrombocytopenia with long-term heparin therapy, which is less common with LMWHs. Both heparin and warfarin increase the risk of retroplacental bleeding during pregnancy, and warfarin-exposed fetuses in the first trimester are at risk for nasal hypoplasia and epiphyseal calcification. As a result, there is no consensus on how to treat anticoagulation in pregnancy.

Bioprosthetic tissue is much less thrombogenic than mechanical valves, and anticoagulation is usually only necessary when there is an arrhythmia. Pregnancy is generally well tolerated if the valve anatomy and left ventricular function are normal and there are no other cardiac abnormalities. When the valve does not work properly, the hazards are increased. Tissue valves deteriorate with age. Mitral bioprostheses degenerate more quickly than aortic bioprostheses, especially in women under the age of 40 years. Women of reproductive age who have bioprosthetic valves may need heart surgery again, which is something to keep in mind when choosing a valve implant before getting pregnant. In the published literature, the rate of endocarditis ranges from 0% to 10%. A detailed evaluation of a pregnant lady with pyrexia and prosthetic valves should be performed to rule out endocarditis. Endocarditis on mechanical prosthetic valves is a sign that the valve has to be replaced. In such cases, prophylaxis against infectious endocarditis is a must. Minimizing the number of vaginal examinations during labor, restricting instrumentation of the genital tract during labor and delivery, paying close attention to antisepsis during labor, ensuring that the placenta is delivered completely, and using prophylactic antibiotics are all ways to reduce the risk of endocarditis.

CONCLUSION

Rheumatic heart disease complicating pregnancy is widespread in underdeveloped nations, necessitating the combined knowledge of professional cardiologists, obstetricians, and anesthesiologists during the pregnancy. Undiagnosed disease may also be discovered for the first time during pregnancy, and the process of giving obstetric care allows for the establishment of postnatal care continuity, with a focus on preventative therapy and contraception.

REFERENCES

1. Khanom M, Hossain A. Valvular heart disease in pregnancy: A review. J Indian Coll Cardiol. 2015;5(3):177-82.
2. Windram JD, Colman JM, Wald RM, Udell JA, Siu SC, Silversides CK. Valvular heart disease in pregnancy. Best Pract Res Clin Obstet Gynaecol. 2014;28(4):507-18.
3. Bhargava B, Agarwal R, Yadav R, Bahl VK, Manchanda SC. Percutaneous balloon aortic valvuloplasty during pregnancy: use of the Inoue balloon and the physiologic antegrade approach. Catheteriz Cardiovasc Diag. 1998;45(4):422-5.
4. Marijon E, Mirabel M, Celermajer DS, Jouven X. Rheumatic heart disease. Lancet. 2012;379(9819):953-64.
5. Otto CM, Nishimura RA, Bonow RO, Carabello BA, Erwin JP 3rd, Gentile F, et al. 2020 AHA/ACC guideline for the management of patients with valvular heart disease: executive summary: a report of the American College of Cardiology/American Heart Association Joint Committee on Clinical Practice Guidelines. Circulation. 2021;143(5):e35-71.
6. Maganti K, Rigolin VH, Sarano ME, Bonow RO. Valvular heart disease: diagnosis and management. Mayo Clin Proc. 2010;85:483-500.
7. Tillquist MN, Maddox TM. Cardiac crossroads: deciding between mechanical or bioprosthetic heart valve replacement. Patient Prefer Adherence. 2011;5:91-9.
8. Salazar E, Izaguirre R, Verdejo J, Mutchinick O. Failure of adjusted doses of subcutaneous heparin to prevent thromboembolic phenomena in pregnant patients with mechanical cardiac valve prostheses. J Am Coll Cardiol. 1996;27(7):1698-703.

CHAPTER 4

Congenital Heart Disease in Pregnancy

CASE SCENARIO

A single ventricle is a relatively uncommon congenital heart defect, accounting for <1% of all congenital heart defects. At the gestational age of 28 weeks, a woman was seen in our obstetric clinic for the first time and discovered to be pregnant with placental bleeding. She also had congenital heart disease and atrial fibrillation, both of which necessitated anticoagulation. With right and left atrioventricular valves entering this chamber and levo-transposition of the great arteries, echocardiography revealed a double-inlet single ventricle with right and left atrioventricular valves entering this chamber. After a thorough conversation with the patient about the risks and advantages of anticoagulation, including the risk of stroke, it was decided to start her on intravenous heparin with close monitoring and keep her pregnant for at least 32 weeks to lower the fetus' postpartum risk. The pregnancy went smoothly, and the patient underwent an elective caesarean surgery at 33 weeks of gestation, resulting in the birth of a healthy baby boy.[1]

INTRODUCTION

Patients with congenital heart disease may decompensate during pregnancy if not able to cope with physiological changes of pregnancy. Complications such as heart failure, arrhythmias, and a worsening of the cardiac condition may raise the risk of morbidity and mortality for both mother and child. When it comes to congenital heart disease, it is frequently detected and treated, and when it comes to planning a pregnancy, counseling and risk prediction are often provided.

COUNSELING

During counseling the following should be discussed:

- The risk for the mother and for the fetus
- Medication use and possible adaptations needed before pregnancy
- The recurrence risk for congenital heart disease in the baby and the long-term outcome for the mother

  Also, reproductive therapies and contraception need attention.

RISK STRATIFICATION

For estimation of maternal complication during and after pregnancy several risk scores have been proposed out of which the modified World Health Organization (WHO) risk classification is important in recognition of risks. This helps in diagnosis and also helps to decide as to who should be referred immediately and who can be evaluated in nontertiary care centers. The WHO categorization appears to function best in women with congenital heart disease, but the addition of clinical factors will allow for a more tailored strategy.[2]

MODIFIED WHO RISK STRATIFICATION (TABLE 1)

The newest European Society of Cardiology (ESC) pregnancy guideline includes a detailed discussion of the classification.

Mild congenital cardiac disease, such as a minor patent ductus arteriosus or mitral valve prolapse, and healed uncomplicated lesions are classified as class I. In comparison to the general pregnant population, these lesions are not associated with a high risk of morbidity or mortality. The risk of pregnancy gradually increases to extremely high risk in Modified WHO class IV which includes women with pulmonary arterial dilatation, severe systemic ventricular dysfunction or severe aortic dilatation.[4,5]

Class I women can be treated in a community hospital, but class IV women are advised not to get pregnant. Women in the mWHO II, II–III, and III classifications are at a modest to moderately higher risk, and evaluation and management throughout pregnancy in a tertiary center is essential.

CLINICAL RISK SCORES

Clinical risk scores are presented in **Table 2**.

PULMONARY ARTERIAL HYPERTENSION

Pulmonary arterial hypertension is classified as mWHO class IV by the WHO. Although the prognosis has improved in the current era of modern medicines, there is still a significant risk of heart failure, ventricular arrhythmias, and higher mortality for the mother. Another reason to be highly restrained is the fetus's dismal outcome. Maternal death ranges from a 28% absolute risk to a little improvement in result in selected patients with congenital cardiac disease, but still a 7% maternal mortality rate. Counseling regarding the high-risk pregnancy and thus the absolute contraindication to pregnancy is still crucial.

Fontan

In women with a Fontan circulation, other reasons than cyanosis also influences the level of risk associated with pregnancy. Higher complication

TABLE 1: Modified WHO classification for maternal cardiac risk.[3]

WHO I	*WHO II*
• Pulmonary stenosis (small/mild) • Patent ductus arteriosus (small/mild) • Mitral valve prolapse (small/mild) • Successfully repaired simple shunt defects (ASD, VSD, PDA, APVR) • **Follow-up during pregnancy:** Once or twice in local hospital • **Delivery:** Local hospital	• Unrepaired ASD or VSD • Repaired tetralogy of Fallot • Turner syndrome without aortic dilatation • **Follow-up during pregnancy:** Every trimester in local hospital • **Delivery:** Local hospital
WHO II-III	*WHO III*
• Mild left ventricular impairment (EF >54%) • Native or tissue valve disease not considered WHO I or IV • Marfan or other HTAD syndrome without aortic dilatation • Aorta <45 mm in bicuspid aortic valve • Repaired coarctation • AVSD • **Follow-up during pregnancy:** Bimonthly in expert centre • **Delivery:** Expert centre	• Left ventricular impairment (30–45%) • Mechanical valve • Systemic right ventricle with good or mildly impaired function • Fontan (if otherwise well) • Unrepaired cyanotic disease • Moderate mitral stenosis • Severe asymptomatic aortic stenosis • Moderate aortic dilatation • **Follow-up during pregnancy:** (bi)monthly in expert centre • **Delivery:** Expert centre
WHO IV: Pregnancy not recommended	
• Pulmonary arterial hypertension • Severe systemic ventricular dysfunction (EF<30%) • Moderate systemic right ventricular dysfunction • Severe mitral stenosis • Severe symptomatic aortic stenosis • Severe aortic dilatation • Vascular Ehlers-Danlos • Severe (re)coarctation • Fontan with any complication • **Follow-up during pregnancy:** Monthly in expert centre • **Delivery:** Expert centre	

(APVR: anomalous pulmonary venous return; ASD: atrial septal defect; AVSD: atrioventricular septal defect; EF: ejection fraction; ESC: European Society of Cardiology; HTAD: hereditary thoracic aorta disease; PDA: persistent ductus arteriosus; VSD: ventricular septal defect; WHO: World Health Organization)

rates are seen mainly with systemic ventricular dysfunction, and significant atrioventricular valve regurgitation and protein-losing enteropathy. Major complications are heart failure, supraventricular arrhythmias, thromboembolic events, and bleeding.

TABLE 2: CARPREG II risk predictors.[6]

Predictor	Points
Prior cardiac events or arrhythmias	3
Baseline NYHA 3-4 or cyanosis	3
Mechanical valve	3
Systemic ventricular dysfunction LVEF <55%	2
High-risk valve disease or left ventricular outflow tract obstruction (aortic valve area <1.5 cm^2, subaortic gradient >30, or moderate to severe mitral regurgitation, mitral stenosis <2.0 cm^2)	2
Pulmonary hypertension, RVSP >49 mm Hg	2
High-risk aortopathy	2
Coronary artery disease	2
No prior cardiac intervention	1
Late pregnancy assessment	1

Primary cardiac event risk: score = 1, 5% risk, score = 2, 10% risk, score = 3, 15% risk, score = 4, 22% risk, and 41% risk if score >4.
(LVEF: left ventricular ejection fraction; NYHA: New York Heart Association; RVSP: right ventricular systolic pressure)

MECHANICAL VALVE

Chances of uncomplicated pregnancy depend upon the balance between thrombotic and bleeding risks, which was about 57% in a large registry of women with a mechanical valve prosthesis.

AORTIC DILATATION

There is increased risk of further dilatation and dissection during pregnancy.

MATERNAL AND FETAL OUTCOME

Pregnancy-induced hypertension (3%), preeclampsia (2%), and postpartum hemorrhage (3%), e.g., do not occur more frequently in women with congenital heart disease in general.

Caesarean sections are usually performed for obstetrical reasons or in high-risk situations such as heart failure, advanced pulmonary hypertension, Eisenmenger syndrome, or early labor when taking oral anticoagulants.

Uteroplacental blood flow is lower in women with congenital heart disease when compared to normal population which results in adverse fetal and neonatal outcome. Fetal mortality (1%), preterm birth (14%), and a low Apgar score are all higher risks for women with congenital heart disease (6%). Neonatal death occurs in 0.5% of all births and is equivalent to the general population, but it is dependent on the mother's underlying congenital condition.

FOLLOW-UP DURING PREGNANCY

- Depending upon the risk stratification the frequency of follow-up is decided. Patients with a low-risk diagnosis can be seen once or twice in a local hospital.
- Evaluation in every trimester is recommended for patients who come under the WHO class II. If the pregnancy is unremarkable, both follow-up and delivery can be done at a local hospital. Women in the WHO classes II–III and higher require at least biweekly follow-up in a dedicated expert center, with the frequency increasing as the WHO class increases.
- In the third trimester, women with cyanosis, pulmonary hypertension, or systemic ventricular failure should be monitored weekly or biweekly.
- A multidisciplinary team composed of at least a cardiologist, obstetrician, and anesthesiologist should devise a delivery strategy.
- Almost all women with congenital heart disease should deliver vaginally with spontaneous labor, with exceptions made for obstetric reasons or in the case of a very high-risk cardiac scenario, as previously mentioned. In general, caesarean section has no advantage over vaginal delivery, and women who have a caesarean section have a lower gestational age and birth weight. All women with congenital heart disease should deliver in a hospital and in moderate-to-complex disease in an expert center.
- Women at risk of abrupt heart failure or arrhythmias may require additional hemodynamic monitoring during birth. Pulse oximetry is the initial phase, which includes continuous heart rate monitoring. Continuous electrocardiogram (ECG) monitoring should be considered in advanced-risk individuals.[7]

REFERENCES

1. Elsherif Z, Mahmood N, Jamil S, Wagas H. Complex congenital heart disease in a complicated and precious pregnancy. BMJ Case Rep. 2015;2015: bcr2015209388.
2. Balci A, Sollie-Szarynska KM, van der Bijl AGL, Ruys TP, Mulder BJ, Roos-Hesselink JW, et al. Prospective validation and assessment of cardiovascular and offspring risk models for pregnant women with congenital heart disease. Heart. 2014;100:1373-81.
3. Risk tools modified WHO (mWHO), CARdiac disease in PREGnancy (CARPREG), Zwangerschap bij Aangeboren HARtAfwijking(ZAHARA), Registry of Pregnancy and Cardiac disease(ROPAC). OR's and rates are dervied from cohorts consisting of approx 60% patients oongenital heart disease (63% in CARPREG II and 58% in ROPAC). Numbers derived from: Silversides et al. JACC, 2018; Drenthen et al., Eur Heart J, 2010; van Hagenet et al., Eur J heart Fail. NYHA, New York Heart Association functional class.OR, Odds Ratio. *Source:* Adapted and modified for congenital heart disease, from ESC 2018 "Cardiovascular diseases during pregnancy (management of) guidelines" Table 3.

4. Regitz-Zagrosek V, Roos-Hesselink JW, Bauersachs J, Blomström-Lundqvist C, Cífková R, De Bonis M, et al. 2018 ESC guidelines for the management of cardiovascular diseases during pregnancy. Eur Heart J. 2018;39:3165-241.
5. Siu SC, Sermer M, Colman JM, Alvarez AN, Mercier LA, Morton BC, et al. Prospective multicenter study of pregnancy outcomes in women with heart disease. Circulation. 2001;104:515-21.
6. Silerslides et al, 2018, with permission from elsevier. Radcliffe Cardiology article Table CARPREG II Risk Predictors Source: US Cardiology review 2018;12(2):119-23.
7. Ruys TPE, Roos-Hesselink JW, Pijuan-Domènech A, Vasario E, Gaisin IR, Iung B, et al. Is a planned caesarean section in women with cardiac disease beneficial? Heart. 2015;101:530-6.

5

CHAPTER

Arrhythmias in Pregnancy

INTRODUCTION

Arrhythmia may present for the first time during pregnancy or maybe an exacerbation of underlying condition. Severe arrhythmias requiring aggressive medical or surgical intervention are rare.

MECHANISM OF ARRHYTHMIA DURING PREGNANCY

Atrial and ventricular myocytes are stretched as a result of increased plasma volume causing early after depolarization, shortened refractoriness, and slowed conduction with activation of stretch activated ion channels. Increase in the size of heart can also sustain reentry more easily as the path length of the potential reentrant circuit is increased. High resting rate is arrhythmogenic and as heart rate is increased in pregnancy it also leads to increased arrhythmogenic potential.[1]

Hormonal and autonomic changes may also contribute to arrhythmias. Hormones such as estrogen and progesterone are known to be proarrhythmogenic. Estrogen also results in increase in number of adrenergic receptors in the myocardium and adrenergic responsiveness.

GENERAL MANAGEMENT ISSUES

It should start by ruling out systemic disorders such as hyperthyroidism and pulmonary embolism. Only arrhythmias causing significant symptoms or hemodynamic compromise which can affect both mother and fetus require treatment. Uncontrolled arrhythmias in a patient should be treated prepregnancy.

Antiarrhythmic Drugs

Most of the drugs used in management of arrhythmias are the Food and Drug Administration (FDA) category C that is the risk to fetus cannot be ruled out on administering these drugs. Main concerning in administering these drugs is the potential risk to the developing fetus, especially between 5 and 10 weeks, where fetus is most sensitive to teratogens. Those with moderate risk but is effective in controlling significant arrhythmias should be continued as the benefits of this outweigh the risks. In the second and third trimesters, point of concern is its effects on fetal growth and development, causing fetal arrhythmias, and effect on uterine contractility. The dose prescribed should be the lowest effective dose.[2]

Electric Cardioversion

When arrhythmias are associated with hemodynamic instability then electric cardioversion is indicated in all stages of pregnancy.[3] Indication for elective use is when arrhythmias are refractory to drugs and does not compromise blood flow to the uterus. Risk of inducing fetal arrhythmia is very small as very small amount of current reaches fetus. There is a risk of initiating preterm labor in later stages of pregnancy. There have been cases of fetal arrhythmias after cardioversion requiring caesarean delivery and hence fetal monitoring is advised.

Catheter Ablation in Pregnancy

Fetal radiation exposure and fetal compromise in the event of maternal hemodynamic instability are the additional risks of this procedure in a pregnant patient. In the event of a complication, the gravid uterus may play a role in difficult patient positioning, performing pericardiocentesis and resuscitation. Part of the procedural planning should include emergency surgical delivery option when this procedure is done in a patient with viable fetus.[4]

MANAGEMENT OF SPECIFIC ARRHYTHMIAS

Palpitations and premature beats palpitations are common during pregnancy which prompt cardiovascular evaluation. Symptomatic patients were treated with cardioselective beta-blockers, preferably after the first trimester of pregnancy.

Supraventricular Tachycardia

The most commonly sustained arrhythmia during pregnancy is supraventricular tachycardia. It is usually well tolerated but in patients with structural heart disease can deteriorate with hemodynamic instability and impaired fetal blood flow.

Atrioventricular Nodal Reentrant Tachycardia

Basic management of atrioventricular nodal reentrant tachycardia (AVNRT) involves avoidance of precipitating factors and use of vagal maneuvers to terminate acute episode. Patients who do not respond to the vagal maneuver are managed with adenosine. In cases which do not respond to adenosine, are given next line of drug which includes intravenous metoprolol or propranolol. Next drug which can be used is verapamil.

In refractory cases with hemodynamically unstable patient with AVNRT during pregnancy have been treated with catheter ablation.

Accessory Pathways and Wolff–Parkinson–White

Arrhythmias during pregnancy are more common in patients with pre-excitation. Intravenous procainamide is the drug of choice. In patients with concealed accessory pathways β-blockers, calcium channel blockers, digoxin, or flecainide may be used for long term. Verapamil or digoxin should not be used in patients with Wolff–Parkinson–White (WPW) because of the risk of rapid accessory pathway conduction during atrial fibrillation (AF). In WPW syndrome, beta-blocker should be used with caution. The treatment of choice for WPW in the nonpregnant patient, this is best avoided if possible during pregnancy.

Atrial Fibrillation and Flutter

Less common during pregnancy are AF with flutter with a prevalence of 2 in 100,000 hospital admissions. Given the increased risk of venous thromboembolism during pregnancy, pulmonary embolism should be ruled out as a cause in any pregnant woman with new-onset AF. Electric cardioversion should be used to treat hemodynamically unstable episodes of AF or flutter. When rate control fails, a rhythm control technique using antiarrhythmic drugs (AADs) is a viable option. In this case, sotalol or flecainide are the preferable AADs.[5]

Systemic anticoagulation should be provided to patients with AF or flutter who have risk factors for thromboembolism.

VENTRICULAR TACHYCARDIA AND SUDDEN CARDIAC DEATH

Ventricular tachycardia (VT) and ventricular fibrillation are rare during pregnancy. Ventricular arrhythmias are most common in people who have structural heart disease and a history of VT. A range of cardiomyopathies, including hypertrophic cardiomyopathy and arrhythmogenic right ventricular cardiomyopathy, have been linked to VT during pregnancy. Peripartum cardiomyopathy should be examined in patients without established structural heart disease who develop symptoms of heart failure in the last month of pregnancy or in the months following birth.

VENTRICULAR TACHYCARDIA IN PREGNANT WOMEN WITHOUT STRUCTURAL HEART DISEASE

Idiopathic VT is usually hemodynamically stable, with a favorable prognosis. It is possible that it will appear for the first time during pregnancy. It is frequently catecholamine sensitive, and in pregnant individuals, therapy of outflow tract VT with cardioselective-blockers is usually beneficial.

LONG QT SYNDROME

Beta-blocker therapy has been linked to a lower risk of cardiac events before, during, and after pregnancy. In women with long QT syndrome and symptoms, beta-blockers should be taken throughout pregnancy and after delivery. Because metoprolol may not be as effective in long QT syndrome 1 and 2, propranolol is preferable.

PREGNANCY AND IMPLANTABLE CARDIOVERTER DEFIBRILLATORS

Implantable cardioverter defibrillator (ICD) implantation may be a good option for pregnant individuals who have unstable ventricular arrhythmias and are at high risk of sudden cardiac death during pregnancy. The safety issues for ICD placement during pregnancy are identical to those addressed in the catheter ablation section. ICDs can be effectively implanted during pregnancy with little or no fluoroscopy if necessary, and some have even done it without it with echocardiographic supervision.

BRADYCARDIA AND CONDUCTION DISORDERS

Congenital total heart block is sometimes discovered during pregnancy for the first time. Because of the risk of bradycardia and syncope with Valsalva, interim pacing during labor and delivery was formerly recommended for all patients with full heart block. Permanent pacing may be required for pregnant women with symptomatic or hemodynamically unstable bradyarrhythmias. Permanent pacemakers, like ICDs, can be effectively installed during pregnancy with minimal amounts of radiation.

CONCLUSION

During the first trimester, therapy should be limited, and medications with the best safety records should be administered initially. Higher-risk techniques should be considered in the case of recalcitrant and life-threatening arrhythmias. Catheter ablation of numerous arrhythmias can be performed with minimum radiation exposure thanks to shielding, sophisticated electroanatomic mapping techniques, and intracardiac echocardiography.

REFERENCES

1. Ninio DM, Saint DA. The role of stretch-activated channels in atrial fibrillation and the impact of intracellular acidosis. Prog Biophys Mol Biol. 2008;97:401-16.
2. Joglar JA, Page RL. Management of arrhythmia syndromes during pregnancy. Curr Opin Cardiol. 2014;29:36-44.
3. Cox JL, Gardner MJ. Treatment of cardiac arrhythmias during pregnancy. Prog Cardiovasc Dis. 1993;36:137-78.
4. Kanjwal Y, Kosinski D, Kanj M, Thomas W, Grubb B. Successful radiofrequency catheter ablation of left lateral accessory pathway using transseptal approach during pregnancy. J Interv Card Electrophysiol. 2005;13:239-42.
5. Camm AJ, Kirchhof P, Lip GY, Schotten U, Savelieva I, Ernst S, et al.; ESC Committee for Practice Guidelines. Guidelines for the management of atrial fibrillation: The task force for the management of atrial fibrillation of the European Society of Cardiology (Esc). Eur Heart J. 2010;12:1360-420.

CHAPTER 6 Peripartum Cardiomyopathy

CASE SCENARIO

A 25-year-old primiparous woman with a history of insulin-dependent diabetes mellitus presented with preeclampsia at 34 weeks of pregnancy and was treated with steroids. Preeclamptic toxemia necessitated an emergency caesarean section at 35 weeks, after which she was discharged home on day 4. She was readmitted with dyspnea and orthopnea 2 days later. Panic attack and pulmonary thromboembolism were the initial differential diagnosis. Only until a chest X-ray revealed pulmonary edema was the diagnosis of decompensated heart failure (HF) made.

She was sent to the National Heart Failure Unit after being intubated. She was kept alive for 5 days by an intra-aortic balloon pump, which she was able to wean off. On her follow-up echocardiogram, her ventricular functions were great. Her beta-blocker, angiotensin-converting enzyme (ACE) inhibitor, and aldosterone antagonist prescriptions are all up to date. She also had a 3-month trial on bromocriptine.

INTRODUCTION

Peripartum cardiomyopathy is defined as idiopathic HF that occurs in the last month of pregnancy or the first 5 months after birth in the absence of any determinable cardiac disease. The quick clinical course of peripartum cardiomyopathy is distinguished by the possibility of spontaneous recovery.[1]

ETIOLOGY

This disease is thought to be idiopathic as any specific causal factors have not yet been identified. Risk factors include multiparity, Black race, maternal age >30 years, twin pregnancies, and history of hypertension, preeclampsia, and eclampsia.

Inflammation's role in peripartum cardiomyopathy—tumor necrosis factor (TNF), interferon-gamma, interleukin-6, C-reactive protein (CRP), and Fas/apoptosis antigen 1 (Apo-1) concentrations in peripartum cardiomyopathy reveal an underlying inflammatory process for the pathophysiologic development of peripartum cardiomyopathy.[2]

Fetal chimerism maternal immune systems destroy the fetal cells escaping into the maternal circulation during pregnancy. Some, however, manage to avoid the weakened maternal immune system throughout pregnancy and settle in the maternal heart, where they remain until the normalized immune system responds postpartum.

Genetic Associations

There may be an overlap in the clinical spectrum of dilated and peripartum cardiomyopathy as suggested by prevalence of similar mutating genes in both.

Current peripartum cardiomyopathy diagnostic criteria:[3,4]

- HF in the last month of pregnancy or 5 months after delivery
- There is no history of cardiac disease
- Unpredictable cause
- The results of an echocardiogram (a, together with b or c; or all of these):
    a. End-diastolic size of the left ventricle >2.7 cm/m^2
    b. M-mode fractional shortening 30%
    c. Ejection fraction of the left ventricle is <0.45

CLINICAL PRESENTATION AND DIAGNOSIS

Majority of cases are seen in first 4 months postpartum and prepartum cases are rare.

Common Symptoms

Dyspnea, cough, orthopnea, hemoptysis, and paroxysmal nocturnal dyspnea are common symptoms. The majority of those who are impacted have a New York Heart Association (NYHA) class III or IV function.

Fatigue, malaise, palpitations, chest and abdominal discomfort, and postural hypotension are other nonspecific symptoms.

Diagnosis

Symptoms may be confused with physiologic changes associated with advanced pregnancy and hence diagnosis requires high degree of suspicion.

Common Signs

Displacement of the apical impulse, presence of S3, and evidence of mitral or tricuspid regurgitation. Other signs which can be seen are engorgement of the neck veins, pedal edema, pulmonary crepitation, and hepatomegaly.

Differential Diagnosis

Obstetric difficulties such as preeclampsia, eclampsia, and amniotic fluid embolism, as well as accelerated hypertension, diastolic dysfunction, systemic infection, pulmonary embolus, electrocardiography, echocardiography, MRI, endomyocardial biopsies, and cardiac protein assays are all used in the diagnosis and monitoring of heart disease.

Electrocardiography there are no pathognomic changes in electrocardiograms. Left ventricular (LV) hypertrophy and ST-T wave abnormalities are commonly seen.

Globally reduced contractility and LV enlargement without hypertrophy are common echocardiographic findings. Mural thrombus, mitral or tricuspid regurgitation, and pericardial effusion can all be diagnosed by echocardiography.

Complications

Complications such as atrial fibrillation and flutter, prolonged PR and QRS intervals, Q wave in anteroseptal leads, and bundle branch blocks are also seen.

FOLLOW-UP

Patients with a high initial left ventricular ejection fraction (LVEF) are less likely to have a future pregnancy recurrence. Prompt echocardiography in all symptomatic pregnant patients can assist identify patients with undiagnosed peripartum cardiomyopathy earlier in the disease's course, allowing for earlier treatment and better outcomes. Patients with a history of peripartum cardiomyopathy can use dobutamine stress echocardiography to measure their contractile reserve and identify individuals who are at risk of return.

Following discharge from the hospital, at 6 weeks and 6 months postpartum, and annually thereafter, follow-up echocardiogram should be performed to assess development.

Cardiac MRI using T2-weighted spin echo sequences aids in the precise diagnosis of myocarditis, necrosis, and LV thrombi, as well as providing correct ventricular volume measures.

Endomyocardial Biopsy Endomyocardial Biopsy

It is a highly specific technique for diagnosing myocarditis.

Cardiac Protein Assays

Cardiac protein assays show promise for diagnosis and postpartum disease monitoring. Other test like cardiac catheterization has been superseded by noninvasive imaging techniques.

MANAGEMENT

- The first line of management is pharmacologic therapy and, if necessary, nonpharmacological therapies.
- Acute event management is by use of oxygen, diuretic, and angiotensin receptor blocker (ARB).
- The second aim is to affect a cure through the administration of targeted therapies.

Diuretics

This lowers preload and alleviates lung congestion and peripheral edema symptoms. During pregnancy and lactation, both hydrochlorothiazide and furosemide are safe. Dehydration caused by diuretics can result in uterine hypoperfusion and metabolic acidosis in the mother, necessitating bicarbonate monitoring and acetazolamide treatment.

Neurohormonal Blockade

First line for management of HF is angiotensin-modulating agents. ACE inhibitors, and angiotensin receptor blockers improve survival but are contraindicated in pregnancy.

Vasodilators

Primary vasodilator drug hydralazine is safe during pregnancy.

Intravenous nitroglycerin starting at 10–20 μg/min and continuing up to 200 μg/min may be required in severe cases.

Inotropic Agents

- Inotropic drugs should only be used in extreme circumstances of poor output, and the patient should be weaned off them as soon as she is hemodynamically stable.
- *Levosimendan:* This medication lowers pulmonary capillary wedge pressure and enhances cardiac output in peripartum cardiomyopathy patients.
- *Digoxin:* During pregnancy, digoxin, an inotropic and dromotropic drug, is safe to take. Due to the scarcity of antepartum medication alternatives and the increasing hemodynamic loads experienced during late pregnancy, digoxin is a popular choice.
- Blockers are prescribed to treat systolic dysfunction.
- *Calcium channel blockers:* Dihydropyridines, such as amlodipine, when used in HF patients are shown to successfully reduce interleukin-6.

Arrhythmia Management

Atrial fibrillation is commonly seen in these patients and digoxin can also be used as first-line therapy. Permanent pacemakers and implantable cardioverter-defibrillators may be required in refractory atrial fibrillation.[5]

Anticoagulation

When LVEF is <0.30 anticoagulation with heparin/Low molecular weight heparin (LMWH) and warfarin is recommended.

Mechanical Circulatory Support and Transplantation

In severe cases, mechanical circulatory support and even heart transplantation may be required. Bridges such as intra-aortic balloon pumps and LV assist devices (LVADs) have been utilized until transplantation is possible.

Immunosuppressive Drugs for Targeted Therapy

Empiric immunosuppressive medication is not suggested because myocarditis does not occur in all instances. When active myocarditis has been verified by endomyocardial biopsy, it should be evaluated for patient care.[6]

Intravenous Immunoglobulin

A new and promising approach for improving cardiac function is intravenous immunoglobulin therapy.

PROGNOSIS IN PERIPARTUM CARDIOMYOPATHY (FIG. 1)

Recovery from peripartum cardiomyopathy is defined as an increase in LVEF of >0.20 or a recovery of LVEF to >0.50%. As previously said, recuperation normally happens between 3 and 6 months after delivery, although it can take up to 48 months. Patients with a delayed diagnosis, a higher NYHA functional

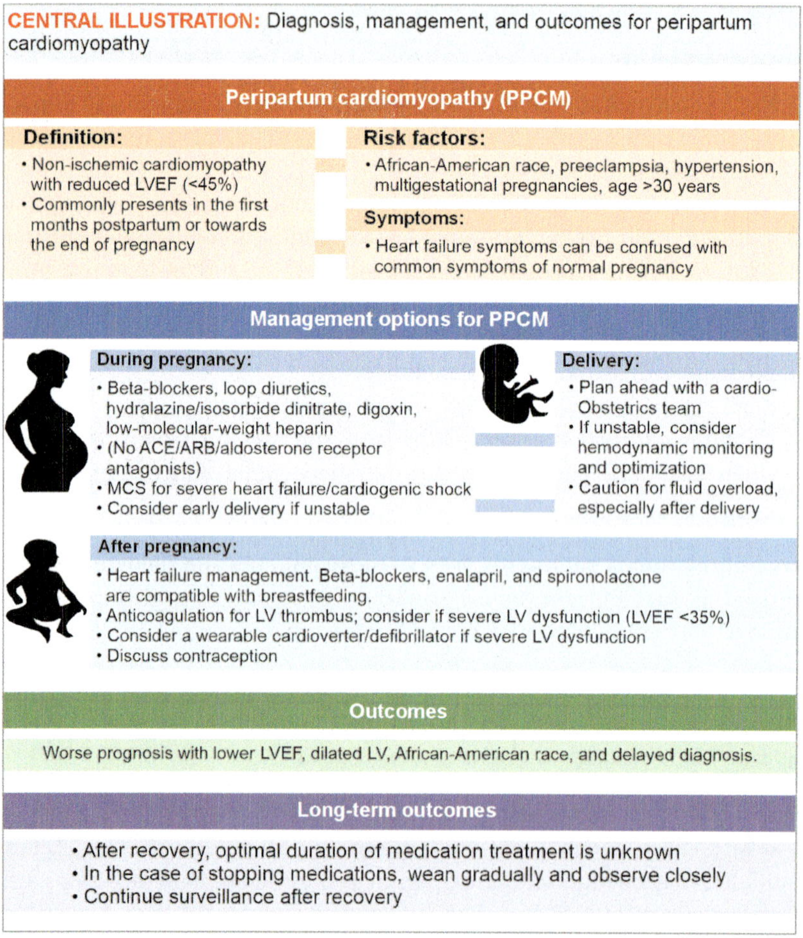

Fig. 1: Diagnosis, management, and outcomes in peripartum cardiomyopathy.[7] (ACE: angiotensin-converting enzyme; ARB: angiotensin receptor blocker; LVEF: left ventricular ejection fraction; MCS: mechanical circulatory support)

Source: Davis MB, Arany Z, McNamara DM, Goland S, Elkayam U. Peripartum Cardiomyopathy: JACC State-of-the-Art Review. J Am Coll Cardiol. 2020;75(2):207-21.

class, black ethnicity, LV thrombus, multiparity, and concurrent medical condition have a slower recovery. It is difficult to anticipate outcomes, and current standards advise against subsequent pregnancies.

CONCLUSION

Peripartum cardiomyopathy is a rare but serious condition of unknown etiology. Diagnosis of peripartum cardiomyopathy requires awareness, high degree of suspicion, and multidisciplinary patient care approach. Management should aim first at improving heart failure symptoms and then at administering targeted therapies.

REFERENCES

1. Mubarik A, Chippa V, Iqbal AM. Postpartum Cardiomyopathy. Treasure Island (FL): StatPearls Publishing; 2022.
2. Bultmann BD, Klingel K, Nabauer M, Wallwiener D, Kandolf R. High prevalence of viral genomes and inflammation in peripartum cardiomyopathy. Am J Obstet Gynecol. 2005;193(2):363-5.
3. Demakis JG, Rahimtoola SH. Peripartum cardiomyopathy. Circulation. 1971;44(5):964-81.
4. Manolio TA, Baughman KL, Rodeheffer R, Pearson TA, Bristow JD, Michels VV, et al. Prevalence and etiology of idiopathic dilated cardiomyopathy (summary of a National Heart, Lung, and Blood Institute workshop). Am J Cardiol. 1992;69(17):1458-66.
5. Midei MG, DeMent SH, Feldman AM, Hutchins GM, Baughman KL. Peripartum myocarditis and cardiomyopathy. Circulation. 1990;81(3):922-8.
6. Isezuo SA, Abubakar SA. Epidemiologic profile of peripartum cardiomyopathy in a tertiary care hospital. Ethn Dis. 2007;17(2):228-33.
7. Mason JW, O'Connell JB, Herskowitz A, Rose NR, McManus BM, Billingham ME, et al. A clinical trial of immunosuppressive therapy for myocarditis. The Myocarditis Treatment Trial Investigators. N Engl J Med. 1995;333(5):269-75.

7

CHAPTER

Pulmonary Artery Hypertension

INTRODUCTION

Pulmonary hypertension (PH) is defined as the rise in mean pulmonary artery pressure (PAP) ≥25 mm Hg at rest as assessed by right heart catheterization (RHC). Pulmonary arterial hypertension (PAH) is characterized by the presence of precapillary PH, defined as a pulmonary artery wedge pressure wedge pressure of ≤15 mm Hg and a pulmonary vascular resistance (PVR) of >3 Wood units. Pregnancy in women with PAH is related to high maternal morbidity and mortality.[1]

Because of the interplay between cardiovascular stressors and complicated physiological changes that occur during pregnancy, as well as the reduced right ventricular (RV) function and aberrant vasculature seen in these patients, preexisting PAH provides a considerable risk of maternal death.[2] There are numerous circulatory changes that occur during pregnancy in order to meet the demands of the fetus and mother. By 32–36 weeks of pregnancy, oxygen consumption has increased by 30%, while blood volume has increased by 40–50%. Cardiac output rises gradually throughout pregnancy beginning in the first trimester and peaks at roughly 28 weeks, almost 50% higher than prepregnancy values. This is a significant difficulty for individuals with PAH who have reduced cardiac function as a result of an increase in RV afterload and cardiac output in response to pressure, whether during exercise or pregnancy. In severe PAH, the resting cardiac output may be <3.0 liters per minute.[3] The cardiovascular needs of pregnancy are not satisfied in certain patients. As the patient strains to meet cardiovascular demands, this is reflected in increased dyspnea or syncope. Early in pregnancy, when further increases in cardiac output are required, the development of these symptoms on minimal exertion or at rest is a worrisome indicator.[4] During pregnancy, a range of hormonal changes occurs, and it is widely believed that pregnancy is a vasodilatory condition. Changes in the secretion of many vasoactive peptides during pregnancy and the postpartum period, on the other hand, may have negative effects on the vasculature, worsening pulmonary vasoconstriction.[5] Rapidly shifting levels of vasoactive constrictors and vasodilators, in particular, during the postpartum period can result in severe pulmonary vasoconstriction, contributing to the high fatality rates found at this time.[6] Physiological changes in pregnancy are explained in the **Flowchart 1**.

Flowchart 1: Physiological changes in pregnancy.[4]

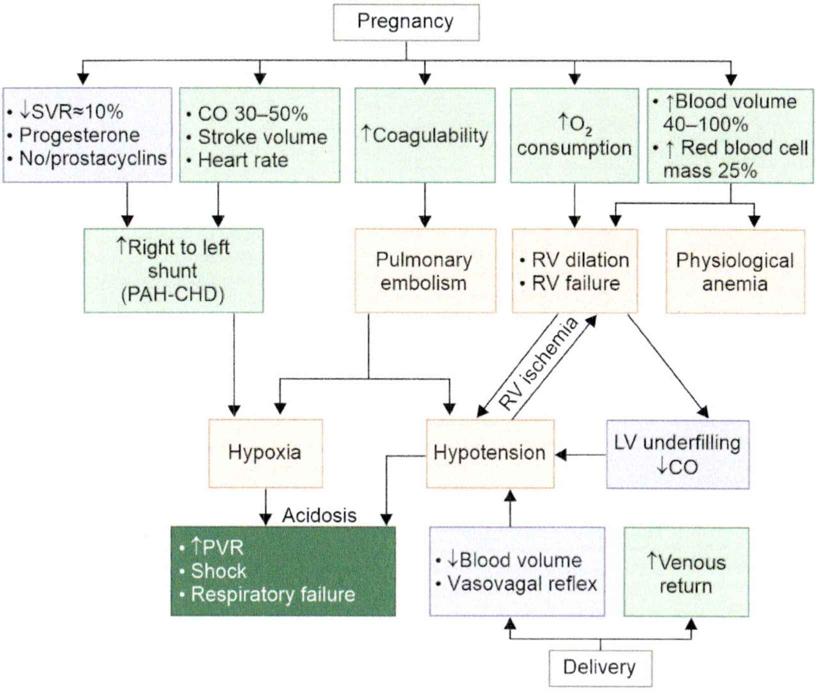

(CHD: congenital heart disease; LV: left ventricular; PAH: pulmonary arterial hypertension; PVR: pulmonary vascular resistance; RV: right ventricular; SVR: systemic vascular resistance)

Source: Yaghi S, Novikov A, Trandafirescu T. Clinical update on pulmonary hypertension. J Investig Med. 2020;68(4):821-7.

Painful uterine contractions cause an extra increase in cardiac output during labor. Analgesia can help to lessen this need. The delivery of the placenta and uterine contractions in the third stage of labor can release up to 500 mL of blood into the circulation. The aorta and venous system are both decompressed after delivery, resulting in an increase in venous return. These may be partially countered by blood losses after delivery, but depending on the impact on the right ventricle, these variations in blood volume may have a detrimental effect on blood pressure. Significant fluid movements after delivery can raise right atrial pressure and have a negative impact on RV function. A negative Starling response resulting from volume-mediated RV dilatation can result in a drastic drop in cardiac output, which can be fatal.[7]

Histological findings from patients with idiopathic pulmonary arterial hypertension (IPAH) show in situ thrombosis, and failure to remove thrombus is a defining feature of chronic thromboembolic pulmonary hypertension (CTEPH). Acute pulmonary thromboembolism (PTE) is more likely to occur

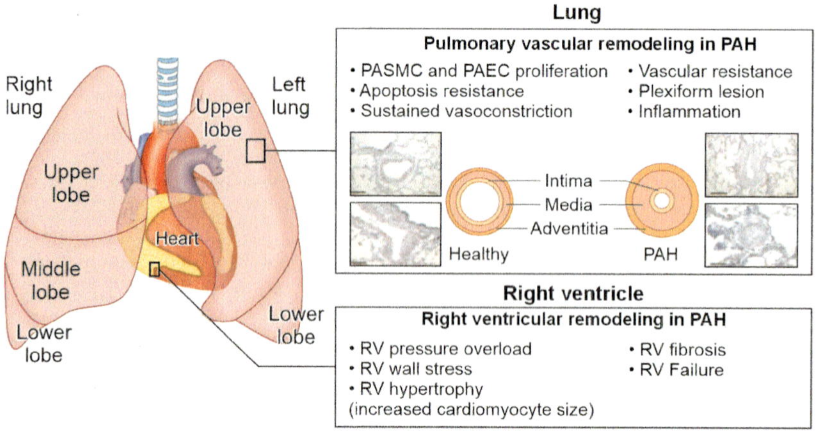

Fig. 1: Pathogenesis of pulmonary artery hypertension.[10] (PAEC: pulmonary arterial endothelial cell; PAH: pulmonary arterial hypertension; PASMC: pulmonary arterial smooth muscle cell; RV: right ventricular)

Source: Bisserier M, Janostiak R, Lezoualc'h F, Hadri L. Targeting epigenetic mechanisms as an emerging therapeutic strategy in pulmonary hypertension disease. Vasc Biol. 2020;2:R17-34.

during pregnancy, especially in patients who have had a caesarean delivery. An increase in afterload occurs when a pulmonary thrombus develops, further decreasing RV function.[8]

Any medical issue that increases the chance of maternal death adds to the stress of dealing with a normal pregnancy for patients and their families. Compliance can be hampered by a variety of factors, especially when dealing with complex medicines and management plans. The paucity of experienced clinicians who can detect small changes in these pregnancies, as well as the lack of randomized controlled trial evidence on how to manage these pregnancies, combine to create a dangerous combination.[9] The pathogenesis of PH is depicted in the **Figure 1**.

HISTORY AND PHYSICAL EXAMINATION

The symptoms of PH are nonspecific and might include chest discomfort, cough, and shortness of breath that is triggered by physical activity. Advanced patients have resting symptoms. Lower extremities edema, dizziness, or syncope are all symptoms of right heart failure.[11] Mechanical problems of PH and aberrant blood flow distribution in the pulmonary vascular bed may be present in some individuals. Hoarseness generated by compression of the left recurrent laryngeal nerve, wheeze caused by massive airway compression, and angina owing to myocardial ischemia induced by compression of the left main coronary artery are among the symptoms associated with pulmonary arterial dilatation. The majority of the symptoms are similar to those of a normal pregnancy.[12]

INVESTIGATIONS

Blood Test

Full blood count, metabolic panel, coagulation studies, and preoperative arterial blood gas must be done. Biomarkers like brain natriuretic peptide (BNP) are useful in monitoring chronic PAH. In the pulmonary embolism, BNP can stratify patients in danger of right ventricular failure (RVF) and troponin I leak may predict mortality.

Electrocardiogram

Electrocardiogram (ECG) may provide supportive evidence of PH, but a normal and standard ECG does not exclude the diagnosis.

Chest Radiograph

At the time of diagnosis, 90% of IPAH patients have an abnormal chest radiograph. Pulmonary arterial dilatation is seen in patients with PAH, in contrast to "pruning" (loss) of the peripheral blood arteries. In more severe cases, the right atrium (RA) and RV expand. The chest radiograph can help in the differential diagnosis of PH by revealing evidence of lung illness or pulmonary venous congestion caused by left heart dysfunction.[13]

Figures 2A and B show features of PH, cardiomegaly (CT ratio >50%) with elevated cardiac apex, enlarged RA, dense bilateral hilum with positive hilum convergence sign, and obliteration of left pulmonary bay.

The gold standard for the diagnosis of PH is true heart or is the right heart or the pulmonary artery catheterization. In resource constrained environment, this is often not necessarily done. RHC directly measures the mean PAP and yields other useful hemodynamic data. For example, it measures

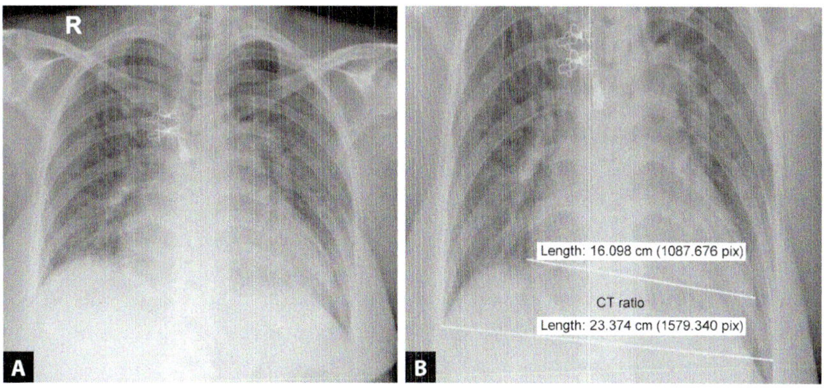

Figs. 2A and B: Chest radiograph suggestive of pulmonary artery hypertension.[14]
Source: Babu V. Pulmonary arterial hypertension. [online] Available from: https://doi.org/10.53347/rID-46751. [Last accessed November, 2024].

the cardiac output and calculates PVR as per Ohm's law. Low CO is a marker of poor prognosis.

Ventilation/perfusion (V/Q) lung scan can be used in the patients with PH to see for chronic thromboembolic PH. CT imaging (high-resolution, contrast-enhanced, and pulmonary angiography) are all available to help provide an important information on vascular, cardiac, parenchymal, and mediastinal abnormalities to find out the cause of PH. Cardiac magnetic resonance (CMR) imaging could also be useful in patients when an ionizing radiation exposure or iodine-based contrast media injection is contraindicated.

PHARMACOLOGICAL MANAGEMENT

The patient's hemodynamic state and illness severity are guided by the diagnosis of the PH type. Thromboembolic events are five times more likely in pregnant women than in nonpregnant women. Patients with group 1 (idiopathic and inheritable PAH) and group 4 (chronic thromboembolic PH) are usually administered anticoagulation for the rest of their lives. Anticoagulation is contentious in women with portal hypertension or Eisenmenger's syndrome because of the danger of bleeding. When taken in the first trimester, vitamin K antagonists have been associated to dose-dependent teratogenesis and an increased risk of fetal cerebral hemorrhage throughout pregnancy. Because unfractionated and low relative molecular weight heparin do not penetrate the placenta, they are safe to use during pregnancy.[15] Because further study on the impact of direct oral anticoagulants (DOACs) in pregnancy is needed, they are categorized as category C medicines. When clinical signs of cardiac failure are present, diuretics (furosemide and hydrochlorothiazide) digoxin and sodium/fluid restriction are recommended. Spironolactone should be avoided because of its association with antiandrogenic effects in male animal fetuses.

Since PH is a rare condition, large-scale studies with long-term follow-up are difficult and expensive to conduct, especially when survival is the primary endpoint. The notion of "hitting hard and hitting early" has been proposed, calling for early dual or triple treatment to slow disease development. Although RHC is required prior to the start of medication therapy, a recent study found that up to 40% of referred patients were already on drug therapy without having completed RHC.[2]

CALCIUM CHANNEL BLOCKERS

Nifedipine, diltiazem, or amlodipine are the mainstays. Mainly reserved for group 1 (PAH) who are vasodilatory responders on RHC. They are contraindicated in nonresponse group (90% of patients). Low cost and widespread availability make them attractive as initial agents. Nonselective pulmonary vasodilators result in systemic side effects, therefore they are not suitable for high-risk patients (WHO class III/IV).

PROSTAGLANDIN ANALOGS

Prostacyclin's are most studied agents and have a proven survival benefit. They produce vasodilatation through a second messenger system, leading to an increased cyclic adenosine monophosphate (cAMP) level.[6]

- *Epoprostenol:* It has very short half-life (<6 minutes) therefore must be infused continuously via a central line. Significant risk of rebound worsening with abrupt/inadvertent interruption of the infusion within 30 minutes.
- *Treprostinil:* 3-hour half-life, intravenous (IV) or subcutaneous (SC) routes of administration. Equivalent efficacy to epoprostenol and stable in a room temperature. Major problem of pain and erythema at the infusion site.
- *Iloprost:* Inhalational route of administration is its main advantage. Because the therapy benefits last just 30–90 minutes after delivery, six to nine nebulizer treatments are required per day (5–15 minutes per treatment). Overall benefits are questionable.

PHOSPHODIESTERASE INHIBITORS

Sildenafil and tadalafil block the phosphodiesterase (PDE)-5 enzyme resulting in an increase in intracellular NO signaling and vasodilation due to an increase in cGMP levels. The fact that it is reasonably inexpensive (in comparison to other PH medicines) is a huge plus, but it is countered by the development of tolerance, which necessitates regular dose adjustments. Sildenafil improved performance in a 6-minute walk test and alleviated the rebound rise in PVR and PAP following the termination of nitric oxide (NO).

INHALED NITRIC OXIDE

Selective pulmonary vasodilator requiring a very dedicated delivery device to administer inhaled nitric oxide (iNO) into ventilator circuit, and this is often not readily available. Risk of accumulation of toxic metabolites necessitating continuous monitoring. It can cause rebound PH after prolong exposure, thus slow weaning and bridging with oral medication is strongly advised.

GUANYLATE CYCLASE STIMULATORS

Riociguat stimulates the soluble enzyme guanylate cyclase, which increases cGMP production inside the cell. It has been approved by the Food and Drug Administration (FDA) for use in inoperable patients with CTEPH and PAH. It improves 6-minute walk distance (6MWD) test, functional class, hemodynamic parameters, and therefore the BNP preform, N-terminal-proBNP (NT-proBNP).

ENDOTHELIN RECEPTOR ANTAGONIST

Endothelin (ET) is a powerful vasoconstrictor and smooth muscle mitogen that may have a role in PAH-related vascular hypertrophy and pulmonary vascular hypertrophy. The ET receptors are blocked by bosentan, ambrisentan, and macitentan, all of which are taken orally. Hemodynamic and functional capacity improvements have been reported.[16] Hepatotoxicity, thrombocytopenia, anemia, and teratogenicity have all been described as side effects. In pregnancy, there is a category X.

CONCLUSION

Pulmonary arterial hypertension (PAH) presents a significant challenge in the context of pregnancy due to its complex interplay with the physiological changes and increased cardiovascular demands that accompany gestation. Women with PAH face considerable risks, including high maternal morbidity and mortality rates, primarily due to the inability of the right ventricle to accommodate increased blood flow and pressure, leading to compromised cardiac output. The adaptations required during pregnancy and the postpartum period can exacerbate the condition, with potential severe outcomes due to pulmonary vasoconstriction and related complications.

Management of PAH in pregnant patients requires a highly cautious, multidisciplinary approach that prioritizes early detection and meticulous cardiovascular monitoring. Pharmacological treatments must be carefully chosen with consideration of their impacts on both mother and fetus, emphasizing the necessity for ongoing research and specialized care protocols to improve outcomes for this vulnerable patient group.

REFERENCES

1. Hoeper MM, Bogaard HJ, Condliffe R, Frantz R, Khanna D, Kurzyna M, et al. Definitions and diagnosis of pulmonary hypertension. J Am Coll Cardiol. 2013;62(25 Suppl):D42-50. doi: 10.1016/j.jacc.2013.10.032. PMID: 24355641.
2. McLaughlin VV, Shah SJ, Souza R, Humbert M. Management of Pulmonary Arterial Hypertension. 2015;65(18):1976-97.
3. Kiely DG, Condliffe R, Wilson VJ, Gandhi SV, Elliot CA. Pregnancy and pulmonary hypertension: a practical approach to management. Obstet Med. 2013;6(4):144-54.
4. Yaghi S, Novikov A, Trandafirescu T. Clinical update on pulmonary hypertension. J Investig Med. 2020;68(4):821-7.
5. Katsuragi S, Yamanaka K, Neki R, Kamiya C, Sasaki Y, Osato K. Maternal Outcome in Pregnancy Complicated With Pulmonary Arterial Hypertension. Cric J. 2012;76(9):2249-54.
6. Elliot CA, Stewart P, Webster VJ, Mills GH, Hutchinson SP, Howarth ES, Bu'lock FA, et al. The use of iloprost in early pregnancy in patients with pulmonary arterial hypertension. Eur Respir J. 2005;26(1):168-73.
7. Zhou Q, Peng P, Liu X, Liu J, Gao J, Chen W. Evaluation of maternal and fetal outcomes in pregnancy complicated with pulmonary arterial hypertension. Ann Palliat Med. 2021;10(2):1404-10.

8. Safdar Z. Pulmonary arterial hypertension in pregnant women. Ther Adv Respir Dis. 2013;7:51-63.
9. Lim K, Chang S, Oh SY, Lee JH, Song J, Kang IS, et al. Pulmonary Arterial Hypertension and Pregnancy: Single Center Experience in Current Era of Targeted Therapy. Korean Circ J. 2019;49(6):545-54.
10. Bisserier M, Janostiak R, Lezoualc'h F, Hadri L. Targeting epigenetic mechanisms as an emerging therapeutic strategy in pulmonary hypertension disease. Vasc Biol. 2020;2:R17-34.
11. Luo J, Shi H, Xu L, Su W, Li J. Pregnancy outcomes in patients with pulmonary arterial hypertension: A retrospective study. Medicine (Baltimore). 2020;99(23):e20285.
12. Chung WK, Austin ED, Best DH, Brown LM, Elliott CG. When to offer genetic testing for pulmonary arterial hypertension. Can J Cardiol. 2015;31(4):544-7. doi: 10.1016/j.cjca.2014.11.005. Epub 2014 Nov 11. PMID: 25840103; PMCID: PMC4418475.
13. Imaging of Pulmonary Hypertension Altschul, Erica et al. CHEST, Volume 156, Issue 2, 211-227.
14. Babu V. Pulmonary arterial hypertension. [online] Available from https://doi.org/10.53347/rID-46751. [Last accessed November, 2024].
15. Chessa M, Brida M, Gatzoulis MA, Diller GP, Roos-Hesselink JW, Dimopoulos K, et al. Emergency department management of patients with adult congenital heart disease: a consensus paper from the ESC Working Group on Adult Congenital Heart Disease, the European Society for Emergency Medicine (EUSEM), the European Association for Cardio-Thoracic Surgery (EACTS), and the Association for Acute Cardiovascular Care (ACVC). Eur Heart J. 2021;42(26):2527-35. doi: 10.1093/eurheartj/ehab272. PMID: 34021343.
16. Olsson KM, Channick R. Pregnancy in pulmonary arterial hypertension. Eur Respir Rev. 2016;25:431-7.

8

CHAPTER

Thromboembolism and Anticoagulation in Pregnancy

INTRODUCTION

Pregnancy is a prothrombotic state and there is fourfold risk of thromboembolism in pregnancy when compared to nonpregnant state. 80% of thromboembolic events in pregnancy are venous and the prevalence ranges from 0.5 to 2.0 per 1,000 pregnant women.[1]

"Thromboembolism in Pregnancy" has high morbidity and mortality hence all pregnant women should be evaluated for risk factors of venous thromboembolism (VTE) in early pregnancy or during prepregnancy counseling.[2]

Pregnancy predisposes to hypercoagulable state increasing the risk of thromboembolic episodes. There is alteration in the levels of coagulation factors.[2] Deep vein thrombosis (DVT) in pregnancy mainly involves the left lower extremity, iliac and iliofemoral veins when compared to nonpregnant women. It is due to increased venous stasis in the left leg, which is caused by the right iliac artery compressing the left iliac vein and the gravid uterus compressing the vena cava. There is increase in the concentrations of many coagulation factors coupled with reduction of many anticoagulation factors. All these factors are responsible for the increased incidence of VTE in pregnancy and immediate postpartum period.[4] **Table 1** states the physiological changes in coagulation system during pregnancy.

RISK FACTORS FOR THROMBOEMBOLISM IN PREGNANCY

There is a higher risk of venous thromboembolic episodes in the in the third trimester. The risk of VTE is higher during the postpartum period than it is during pregnancy, especially during the first week postpartum.[2]

For VTE in pregnancy, most important individual risk aspect is a personal history of thrombosis. The risk of recurrent VTE during pregnancy is increased threefold to fourfold and 15–25% of all cases of VTE in pregnancy are recurrent events. **Table 2** states the risk factors for thromboembolism in pregnancy.

TABLE 1: Physiological changes in coagulation system during pregnancy.[5]

Coagulation factor	*Change from nonpregnant state*
Antithrombin III	No change
Plasma fibrinogen (factor 1)	↑
Factor II	No change
Factor V	No change
Factor VII	↑
Factor VIII	↑
Factor IX	No change
Factor X	↑
Free protein S	↓
Plasminogen activator inhibitor 1	↑
Plasminogen activator inhibitor 2	↑
Protein C	No change
von Willebrand factor	↑

Source: Moore L, Pereira N. Physiological changes of pregnancy. In: Velde M, Scholefield H, Plante L (Eds). Maternal Critical Care: A Multidisciplinary Approach. Cambridge: Cambridge University Press; 2013. pp. 107-1.

TABLE 2: Risk factors for thromboembolism in pregnancy.[3]

1. ***Preexisting risk factors:***	
Previous VTE (except a single event related to major surgery)	4
Previous VTE provoked by major surgery	3
Known high-risk thrombophilia	3
Medical comorbidities, e.g., cancer, heart failure; active systemic lupus erythematosus, inflammatory polyarthropathy or inflammatory bowel disease; nephrotic syndrome; type I diabetes mellitus with nephropathy; sickle cell disease; and current intravenous drug user	3
Family history of unprovoked or estrogen-related VTE in first-degree relative	1
Known low-risk thrombophilia (no VTE)	1a
Age (>35 years)	1
Obesity	1 or 2b
Parity ≥3	1
Smoker	1
Gross varicose veins	1

Contd...

Contd...

2. ***Obstetrics risk factors:***	
Preeclampsia in current pregnancy	1
ART/IVF (antenatal only)	1
Multiple pregnancy	1
Caesarean section in labor	2
Elective caesarean section	1
Midcavity or rotational operative delivery	1
Prolonged labor (>24 hours)	1
PPH (>1 l or transfusion)	1
Preterm birth < 37^{+0} weeks in current pregnancy	1
Stillbirth in current pregnancy	1
Any surgical procedure in pregnancy or puerperium except immediate repair of the perineum, e.g., appendicectomy, postpartum sterilization	3
Hyperemesis	3
OHSS (first trimester only)	4
Current systemic infection	1
Immobility and dehydration	1

(ART: assisted reproductive technology; IVF: in vitro fertilization; OHSS: ovarian hyperstimulation syndrome; PPH: postpartum hemorrhage; VTE: venous thromboembolism)
Source: Goecke T, Voigt F, Rath W. Thromboprophylaxis following cesarean section–a nation-wide survey from Germany (Green top guidelines no. 37.). J Matern Neonatal Med. 2020;33(14):2359-65.

RISK ASSESSMENT FOR VENOUS THROMBOEMBOLISM (BOX 1)

BOX 1: Risk assessment for venous thromboembolism (VTE).[3]

- If total score ≥4 antenatally, consider thromboprophylaxis from the first trimester.
- If total score is 3 antenatally, consider thromboprophylaxis from 28 weeks.
- If total score ≥2 postnatally, consider thromboprophylaxis for at least 10 days.
- If admitted to hospital antenatally consider thromboprophylaxis.
- If prolonged admission (≥3 days) or readmission to hospital within the puerperium consider thromboprophylaxis.

For patients with an identified bleeding risk, the balance of risks of bleeding and thrombosis should be discussed in consultation with a haematologist with expertise in thrombosis and bleeding in pregnancy.

Source: Goecke T, Voigt F, Rath W. Thromboprophylaxis following cesarean section—a nation-wide survey from Germany (Green top guidelines no. 37.). J Matern Neonatal Med. 2020;33(14):2359-65.

CLINICAL DIAGNOSIS

There is difference in the clinical features of DVT in pregnancy women as compared to nonpregnant patient with respect to lateralization and extent.

In 9 out of 10 of cases, left leg is affected and the proximal veins are affected most commonly. But in the nonpregnant women, DVT is limited to the calf veins which is rare during pregnancy but may occur in the postpartum period. There are a very few differential diagnoses of a painful, swollen lower limb in pregnancy, and other cases such as ruptured Baker's cyst and hematomas do not occur commonly in this age group. Cellulitis is also rare and can be diagnosed easily by history and clinical features.[5,6] In case of superficial thrombophlebitis, the pain, swelling, erythema, and tenderness are localized but it may lead to DVT. Clinical feature of DVT includes lower leg edema, muscle cramping, and is always unilateral. It is associated with pain on compression of the calf or on deep palpation in the femoral triangle. Homan's sign is said to be positive when dorsiflexion of the foot causes pain but it is nonspecific. Sometimes feature of DVT is preceded by severe low back pain.

DVT can occur at other sites which is very rare and may affect the upper limb or splanchnic veins. The symptoms of pulmonary embolism include chest pain which is acute in onset, and dyspnea may be associated with hemoptysis and low-grade fever.[7]. The diagnosis is often delayed. The differential diagnosis includes chest infection with pleurisy and pneumothorax, but as a rule, pulmonary infarction should be considered most likely until it has been excluded or an alternative diagnosis identified. Women present with only dyspnea and may lead to a diagnostic challenge. In case of a large embolus, the dyspnea is severe and is sudden in onset associated with oxygen desaturation.[8] The features of right heart failure start manifesting such as raised jugular venous pressure. In severe cases along with dyspnea and cyanosis, hypotension occurs leading to collapse or sudden death. There may be absence of chest pain or central chest pain because of myocardial infarction resulting from increased right ventricular work due to low arterial oxygen tension.[9] There should be high-value suspicion otherwise crucial time may be lost in making the diagnosis and ruling out other nonsignificant causes.

INVESTIGATIONS

Ultrasonography

Ultrasonography is a noninvasive and sensitive test. Diagnostic features include lack of vessel compressibility, absence of blood flow, and vessel dilation or visualization of the thrombus. But, there is low sensitivity for thrombus confined to the distal calf veins. But, isolated distal calf vein thrombus is very rare and risk of embolization.[10] In case of doubt, repeat ultrasonography may be required.

Magnetic Resonance Imaging

It is sensitive to the presence of DVT. Its role remains uncertain and contraindications to use of some contrast media require consideration.

X-ray Contrast Venography

X-ray contrast venography with shielding of the uterus is a rarely required option. It is invasive, causes some discomfort, and inevitably involves radiation exposure, but the diagnostic sensitivity is high.

Arterial Blood Gas

Arterial blood gas analysis is used to indicate the degree of hypoxia, but may be normal in pulmonary infarction.

Computed Tomography Scan

Computed tomography (CT) scan of the chest is thought to have the greatest sensitivity for pulmonary embolus among noninvasive tests. CT angiography may be a preferred approach, although technical limitations in pregnancy have been identified. Radiation scatter to the abdomen is sufficiently low to be considered safe for use in pregnancy.

D-dimer

D-dimer is a product of the plasmin digestion of cross-linked fibrin. An increased concentration in plasma is a marker for thrombus formation. Although this test is sensitive, it is not specific for VTE and is insufficient to confirm the diagnosis. Further, diagnostic algorithms that use a D-dimer assay were validated only in previously healthy, nonpregnant, nonhospitalized subjects. Products of fibrin digestion increase in concentration in plasma from approximately 10 weeks' gestation in healthy pregnancy and increase further and abruptly immediately postpartum.[11]

TREATMENT

Most clinicians consider low-molecular weight heparin (LMWH) the anticoagulant of choice. LMWH is administered by subcutaneous injection at the recommended dose for the particular product based on early pregnancy body weight. Once daily administration may be preferred for convenience and is reasonable as long as therapeutic levels can be maintained.[11] Coagulation times, such as activated partial thromboplastin time (aPTT), are not appropriate for this purpose because the aPTT may remain short, even in patients who are given therapeutic doses of LMWH. The anti-Xa assay gives an indication of the pharmacologic response but is a poor predictor of antithrombotic efficacy and provides limited information on bleeding risk in nonpregnant subjects. A peak (4-hours after injection) plasma anti-Xa concentration of around 0.5–1.0 anti-Xa international units appears to be acceptable for a 12-hourly regimen, with slightly higher peak levels sought for a 24-hourly regimen.[12]

There are few indications for use of unfractionated heparin (UFH) rather than LMWH in the context of VTE. It may, however, be justified if there is concern that rapid reversal of the anticoagulant effect may be unpredictably and urgently required, in renal failure, and in the initial management of unstable pulmonary embolism. Whether UFH or LMWH is administered in treatment doses, the platelet count should be monitored from day 5 until around day 20. A progressive, unexplained decrease in the platelet count suggests heparin-induced thrombocytopenia. In the event of this rare complication, heparin should be discontinued. The condition is caused by the development of platelet-activating antibody, and there is a high risk of further thrombosis if the heparin is continued. Warfarin does not appear to be effective for the prevention of thrombosis in this situation. Lepirudin, a direct inhibitor of thrombin, is the alternative anticoagulant of choice in nonpregnant patients with heparin-induced thrombocytopenia, and there are occasional reports of its use in pregnancy. Another alternative is the heparin-like danaparoid, but cross-reactivity may be a problem and there have been problems with availability.[13] It has been used in pregnancy. Fondaparinux can be considered as an alternative.

The initial management of most cases of pulmonary embolism is comparable with that of DVT. The exception is life-threatening massive pulmonary embolism, in which the relative risks of surgical embolectomy and thrombolytic therapy must be considered urgently. Elevating the affected limb helps to relieve symptoms in DVT, and analgesia is recurrently necessary because of the substantial swelling and discomfort caused by either proximal venous occlusion or the pain related with pulmonary infarction. Confinement to bed is not mandatory. Fitted (vs. one size fits all) graduation compression stockings should be used as soon as resolution of swelling allows them to be worn without discomfort. Full-dose heparin treatment should be maintained to delivery. The patient should be advised to withhold the next due dose of heparin once labor has begun or the morning of a planned induction.[14] There has been some concern about the safety of spinal or epidural anesthesia in laboring women who are receiving anticoagulants. In general, insertion and withdrawal of a spinal catheter should be avoided within 12 hours of a subcutaneous dose of LMWH, and preferably for 24 hours after a treatment dose. Whether the risk is increased after this period is unclear, but the potential risk must be balanced against the needs for analgesia and anesthesia during labor.

If no abnormal bleeding occurs during delivery, heparin can be reintroduced 12–24 hours postpartum. Alternatively, warfarin may be initiated along with heparin (until the INR is in the therapeutic range, when heparin can be discontinued) and continued postpartum. Anticoagulation is typically continued 6–12 weeks postpartum or a total of 3 months from the initial diagnosis of VTE, whichever is longer. Although warfarin is secreted in breast milk, the breastfed neonate of a treated mother is not adversely affected. However, warfarin is best avoided when the mother is expressing milk to feed to a severely premature neonate.[15]

THROMBOPROPHYLAXIS IN PREGNANCY (FIG. 1)

Thromboprophylaxis should be offered selectively. All pregnant women should undergo clinical assessment for risk of VTE. Population screening for hereditary thrombophilia is not performed as a routine and should be based on the clinical circumstances and the family history. When a heritable thrombophilia is detected in an asymptomatic subject as part of a family study, this information can be used for an informed risk assessment. Acquired factors are at least as important as genetic predisposition in assessing thrombotic risk. A personal history of VTE is an important consideration for thromboprophylaxis in pregnancy.[2] In addition, patient's age, parity, and weight can be considered. Limited mobility and some chronic medical conditions such as systemic lupus erythematosus may be relevant.

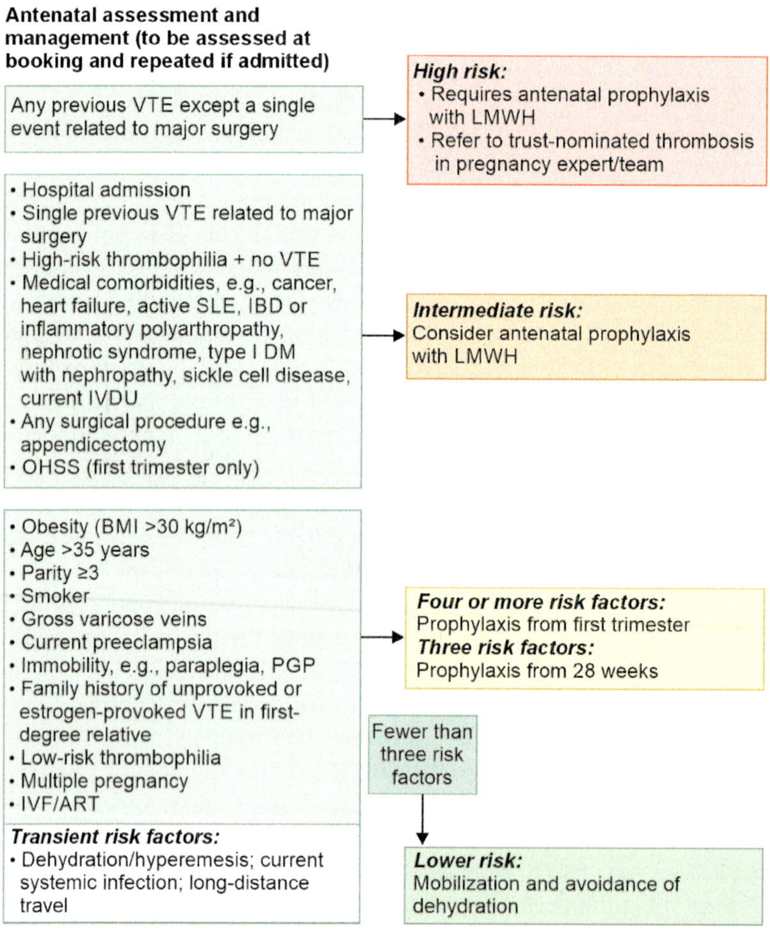

Fig. 1

Contd....

Contd....

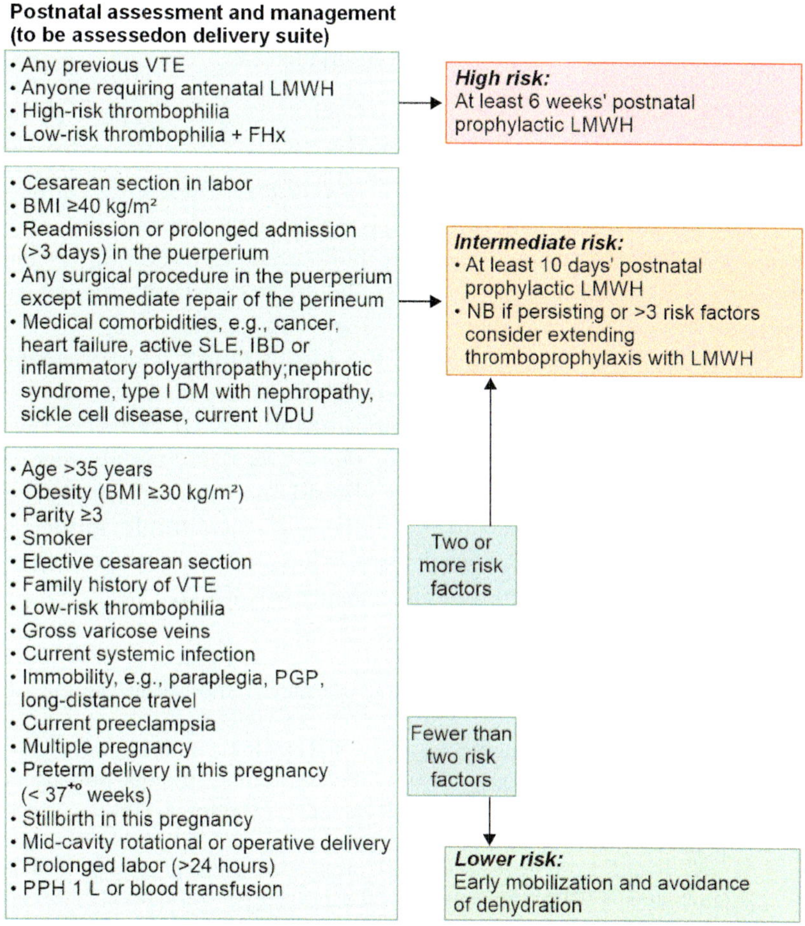

Antenatal and postnatal prophylactic dose of LMWH
Weight <50 kg = 20 mg enoxaparin/2,500 units dalteparin/3,500 units tinzaparin daily
Weight 50–90 kg = 40 mg enoxaparin/5,000 units dalteparin/4,500 units tinzaparin daily
Weight 91–130 kg = 60 mg enoxaparin/7,500 units dalteparin/7,000 units tinzaparin daily
Weight 131–170 kg = 80 mg enoxaparin/10,000 units dalteparin/9,000 units tinzaparin daily
Weight >170 kg = 0.6 mg/kg/day enoxaparin/75 u/kg/day dalteparin/75 u/kg/day tinzaparin

Fig. 1: Obstetric thromboprophylaxis risk assessment and management of venous thromboembolism (VTE).[3]
Source: RCOG. Royal College of Obstetricians and Gynaecologists. (2015). Thromboembolic Disease in Pregnancy and the Puerperium: Acute Management (Green-top Guideline No. 37b). [online] Available from: https://www.rcog.org.uk/globalassets/documents/guidelines/gtg-37b.pdf [Last accessed Nov., 2024].

The risk of venous thrombosis is greatest in the puerperium and higher yet in women who have had caesarean delivery, especially as an emergency procedure or in preeclampsia. The RCOG in the United Kingdom has recommended an algorithm, based on an assessment of personal and family history, heritable thrombophilia, and acquired risk factors. Postpartum thromboprophylaxis with heparin or warfarin should be given. Expert review of risk factor assessment is strongly recommended.[3]

CONCLUSION

Pregnancy significantly enhances the risk of venous thromboembolism (VTE), making it a critical concern for maternal healthcare. Due to physiological changes, pregnant women experience a hypercoagulable state, which escalates the risk of thrombotic events, particularly in the venous system, primarily affecting the lower extremities and, more commonly, the left side due to anatomical and physiological alterations during pregnancy.

Thorough risk assessment is essential, ideally during early pregnancy or prepregnancy counseling, to identify those at elevated risk. This includes women with a personal or family history of VTE, as well as those with other contributing factors such as obesity, age, and certain medical conditions. Management strategies should incorporate appropriate thromboprophylaxis tailored to the individual's risk profile, guided by comprehensive clinical guidelines. The use of low-molecular-weight heparin (LMWH) remains a cornerstone in the management of VTE.

REFERENCES

1. James AH. Venous thromboembolism in pregnancy. Arterioscler Thromb Vasc Biol. 2009;29(3):326-31.
2. American College of Obstetricians and Gynecologists' Committee on Practice Bulletins—Obstetrics. ACOG Practice Bulletin No. 196: Thromboembolism in Pregnancy. Obstet Gynecol. 2018;132(1):e1-e17. Erratum in: Obstet Gynecol. 2018;132(4):1068.
3. RCOG. Royal College of Obstetricians and Gynaecologists. (2015). Thromboembolic Disease in Pregnancy and the Puerperium: Acute Management (Green-top Guideline No. 37b). [online] Available from https://www.rcog.org.uk/globalassets/documents/guidelines/gtg-37b.pdf [Last accessed Nov., 2024].
4. Bates SM, Rajasekhar A, Middeldorp S, McLintock C, Rodger MA, James AH, et al. American Society of Hematology 2018 guidelines for management of venous thromboembolism: venous thromboembolism in the context of pregnancy. Blood Adv. 2018;2(22):3317-59.
5. Moore L, Pereira N. Physiological changes of pregnancy. In: Velde M, Scholefield H, Plante L (Eds). Maternal Critical Care: A Multidisciplinary Approach Cambridge: Cambridge University Press; 2013. pp. 107-19.
6. Goecke T, Voigt F, Rath W. Thromboprophylaxis following cesarean section–a nation-wide survey from Germany. J Matern Neonatal Med. 2020;33(14): 2359-65.
7. Kolettis D, Craigo S. Thromboprophylaxis in Pregnancy. Obstet Gynecol Clin North Am. 2018;45(2):389-402.

8. Nichols KM, Henkin S, Creager MA. Venous Thromboembolism Associated With Pregnancy: JACC Focus Seminar. J Am Coll Cardiol. 2020;76(18): 2128-41.
9. Chan WS. Venous thromboembolism in pregnancy. Expert Rev Cardiovasc Ther. 2010;8(12):1731-40.
10. American College of Obstetricians and Gynecologists' Committee on Practice Bulletins-Obstetrics. ACOG Practice Bulletin No. 197: Inherited Thrombophilias in Pregnancy. Obstet Gynecol. 2018;132(1):e18-e34. Erratum in: Obstet Gynecol. 2018;132(4):1069.
11. Marik PE. Venous thromboembolism in pregnancy. Clin Chest Med. 2010;31(4):731-40.
12. Abe K, Kuklina EV, Hooper WC, Callaghan WM. Venous thromboembolism as a cause of severe maternal morbidity and mortality in the United States. Semin Perinatol. 2019;43(4):200-4.
13. Abu-Shaheen A. Pregnancy and Venous Thromboembolism: Risk Factors, Trends, Management, and Mortality. Biomed Res Int. 2020;2020:4071892.
14. Villani M, Ageno W, Grandone E, Dentali F. The prevention and treatment of venous thromboembolism in pregnancy. Expert Rev Cardiovasc Ther. 2017;15(5):397-402.
15. Ralli E, Zezza L, Lillo R, Conti E, Comito C, Caserta D, et al. Tromboembolismo venoso in gravidanza: attuale stato dell'arte [Venous thromboembolism in pregnancy: current state of the art]. Minerva Med. 2013;104(5):563-78.

9

CHAPTER

Ischemic Heart Diseases

INTRODUCTION

Pregnancy causes significant hemodynamic changes, which may increase the risk of infarction in patients with undiagnosed coronary artery disease. By the early to mid-trimester, there has been a 50% increase in intravascular volume, with the increased plasma volume providing extra stress and perhaps aggravating ischemia.[1] A 30–50% increase in stroke volume is linked to increased plasma volume. During pregnancy, the cardiac output rises by 40–60%. The cardiac output rises by around 25% in the first trimester, 50% in the second trimester, and up to 80% in the third trimester. During labor, cardiac output has been shown to increase, with up to 500 mL being pumped into intravascular space.[2] During delivery, an autotransfusion may occur, followed by a drop in cardiac output, which has been associated to postpartum hemorrhage and vena caval hypertension.[3] Pregnancy can cause a relative hypercoagulable condition, which worsens as the pregnancy progresses and peaks at or around delivery and in the early postpartum period.

CLASSIFICATION OF ISCHEMIC HEART DISEASES

In general, ischemic heart disease (IHD) is divided into two categories: (1) Angina pectoris (also known as transitory myocardial ischemia) and (2) myocardial infarction (MI) (also known as Angina pectoris).[4]

Angina pectoris: Angina pectoris, in all of its forms, is quite uncommon in pregnancy, with only a few occurrences documented. Angina pectoris is not present in the majority of pregnant women who have an MI. Despite the rarity of angina pectoris during pregnancy, those who develop it are considered to be at a high risk of future MI and should be treated accordingly.

Myocardial infarction: In pregnancy, myocardial infarction can cause a variety of symptoms. Typically, the patient may complain of acute central chest discomfort that radiates to the jaw and moves to the left arm. The discomfort is also linked to fainting or may be collapsing; the patient becomes highly nervous, sweats profusely, and may have nausea and vomiting.

PREDISPOSING FACTORS

Smoking, maternal age, family hyperlipidemia, hypertension, and diabetes are all risk factors for MI. Pregnancy is linked to an increased risk of developing hypertension (preeclampsia and eclampsia), as well as the aggravation of preexisting essential or secondary hypertension. A history of high blood pressure was discovered in one-third of the instances of MI in pregnancy that were reported.[5]

In pregnancy, there are many risk factors for IHD. When examining pregnant women with suspected IHD, it is crucial to get a complete medical history, since most studies show that most women with AMI during pregnancy have at least one underlying risk factor for coronary artery disease (CAD), and many have several risk factors.[6] Preeclampsia and hypertension have long been linked to cardiovascular illness later in life, but new research suggests that pre-eclampsia is linked to a higher risk of acute myocardial infarction (AMI), which is most noticeable during the puerperium. Hypertension is also linked to AMI and pregnancy because it may worsen damage to blood vessels that have already experienced negative remodeling as a result of pregnancy's hemodynamic stress and endothelial activation.[7]

THE DIAGNOSIS OF MYOCARDIAL INFARCTION IN PREGNANCY: CLINICAL PRESENTATION

Excruciating retrosternal chest pain radiating to the left shoulder is a common presenting sign of MI. The severity of the pain and diaphoresis (sweating), which is generally linked with myocardial ischemia/infarction, is essential in distinguishing MI discomfort from other types of chest pain associated with pregnancy. The physical examination of a patient with an AMI is nonrevealing. Occasionally, cardiac murmurs can be heard, although they are seldom diagnostic or helpful. The presence of pulmonary edema and cardiac failure are both hallmarks of a severe MI and indicate a poor prognosis.[8]

LABORATORY INVESTIGATION

Diagnosing CAD during pregnancy is difficult and may be dangerous to the baby. Noninvasive procedures that represent the least level of harm to the fetus should be used initially if at all feasible. Exertion electrocardiography has a lesser accuracy in identifying coronary artery disease in women than in men, and fetal bradycardia has been documented in healthy women during maximum exercise. As a result, for the assessment of ischemic cardiac disease during pregnancy, a submaximal exercise program with fetal monitoring is frequently indicated.[5] Because of the risk of teratogenesis, nuclear imaging should be avoided throughout organogenesis (10–50 days). Nuclear imaging may still cause prenatal growth retardation, central nervous system abnormalities, and perhaps an increased risk of cancer in the second and third trimesters. Stress echocardiography may be a viable method for determining ischemia and left ventricular function during pregnancy, as well as in individuals with established or suspected coronary artery disease.[9]

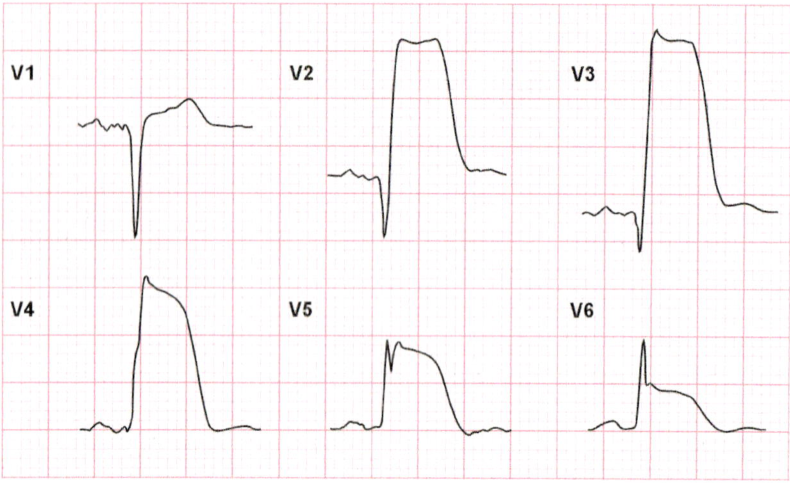

Fig. 1: Anterior myocardial infarction with gross ST segment elevation (showing "tombstone" R waves).[10]
Source: Morris F, Brady WJ. ABC of clinical electrocardiography: Acute myocardial infarction-Part I. BMJ (Clin res ed.). 2002;324(7341):831-4.

Cardiac catheterization has dangers as well, though it is safe to do during pregnancy. Reduce fetal radiation exposure by using appropriate abdominal shielding, a brachial or radial approach, and shorter fluoroscopy periods. Exposure to <10 radicals is considered minimal risk, while exposure to >15 radicals poses a serious danger to the fetus. Cardiac catheterization should only be utilized during pregnancy if other diagnostic options are insufficient or inappropriate. It is likely that the diagnosis of AMI is not suspected as often because it should be within MI and has a low degree of suspicion in general, and its signs and symptoms are frequently misdiagnosed as normal pregnant symptoms.[11]

Electrocardiography and variations in cardiac enzyme levels are used to confirm the diagnosis of AMI in pregnant patients, just as they are in nonpregnant individuals. Normal pregnancy may show left- or right-axis deviation, a minor Q wave in lead III, T wave inversion, or an elevated R/S ratio in leads V1 and V2, making electrocardiographic identification of ischemia more difficult. During caesarean (C)-section, ST segment depression has been documented, which mimics myocardial ischemia but is unrelated to wall motion anomalies.[12] The level of cardiac troponin is recommended above other cardiac indicators for measurement. Troponin levels are not affected by uterine contractions or cell breakdown during labor and delivery, which may lead to significant increases in myoglobin, creatine kinase, and creatine-kinase MB levels. Although it is not a definite diagnostic for ischemia, echocardiography is helpful in assessing wall motion.

MANAGEMENT

An obstetrician, cardiologist, anesthesiologist, dietitian, and a social welfare professional should all be involved in the care of IHD during pregnancy. This team should work together to assist the patient in identifying and preventing risk factors for recurrent ischemia and infarction, recognizing the progression of ischemia to infarction, implementing appropriate monitoring systems, and educating the patient about the condition's potential consequences. The difficulties of abortion in early pregnancy for the management of a patient with IHD is debatable. The evidence that a pregnancy termination reduces the risk of a myocardial ischemic infarction patient is uncertain. However, in the case of a patient with increasing ventricular failure, pregnancy termination may be a better alternative.

GENERAL MEASURES

In the case of a symptomatic patient, bedrest might help to reduce oxygen demand. During acute episodes, patients should be given oxygen supplements. Controlling pain in patients who have had infarction is a critical part of their treatment. Analgesia should be administered intravenously and is capable of decreasing or eliminating pain. Anxiety and tension may be reduced as a result of pain reduction. The drug of choice is morphine (risk category C).

Morphine reduces preload via increasing venous pooling, in addition to its strong analgesic impact. Morphine should be given intravenously since it has a faster impact and prevents the release of muscle enzymes at the injection site, which might cause problems when interpreting cardiac enzyme profiles. Providing emotional and psychological assistance to the patient to alleviate worry may minimize the occurrence of MI or prevent the current one from worsening. Delivery should be postponed in patients who have had the AMI in late pregnancy. A patient with an acute infarct should, ideally, be undelivered for at least a fortnight after the stroke has occurred. The mortality rate can be reduced by at least 15% by extending the time between the infarct and delivery, from 50 to 35% or less. This is a crucial clinical point since the occurrence of an infarct might cause the obstetric team to become anxious about delivering the patient.[10,13]

The lateral recumbent posture is the best position for giving birth. This posture prevents vena caval compression and the resulting reduction in venous return. Improved cardiac contractility, maintained coronary blood flow, and reduced myocardial oxygen demand are other signs of venous return stability.[5] A patient in labor who has had the AMI should be treated in the coronary ICU. Because these patients are at risk of AMI progression and fatal dysrhythmias, they should be treated in a setting where they can get prompt and adequate treatment. Because the fetus is usually unaffected by maternal MI, the major focus should be on the mother rather than the fetus.

Continuous pregnancy monitoring in the hospital is typically advised for patients with MI. The postinfarction treatment should include a careful and regular examination for signs and symptoms of heart failure and/or ventricular dysrhythmias. The role of antiarrhythmic medications in prophylaxis is debatable. Prophylaxis is not recommended for patients with simple MI who do not have severe dysrhythmia. Intravenous prophylaxis is recommended for patients who suffer from temporary or persistent dysrhythmias.[13]

The cardiologist should start antiarrhythmic therapy after consulting with the obstetrician. In the case of the MI, intravenous lidocaine (risk category B) is the medication of choice for treating acute dysrhythmias. In patients with AMI, heart failure characterized by worsening peripheral and pulmonary edema may be a medical emergency. It is advised that furosemide is used to reduce intravascular volume. Patients who have had the MI are more likely to develop thromboembolic illness. Because of the hypercoagulable condition that occurs during pregnancy, this risk may be exacerbated.

Prophylactic heparin should be started as a result. For unfractionated heparin, low-molecular weight, the optimum dosage is 5,000–10,000 SC bid. Despite the fact that heparin, such as enoxaparin 40 mg bid (risk category C), has a long half-life and a potential risk of bleeding if the patient starts laboring within a few hours of treatment, it will be utilized. Full heparinization is required in patients with an intramural thrombus, whether suspected or confirmed.[14]

SPECIFIC MEASURES

Surgical and medical interventions are used in the treatment of individuals who have had the AMI. Nitroglycerine (risk category B) can be administered orally, sublingually, intravenously, or through a dermal patch to patients with AMI. The coronary arteries widen in the presence of nitroglycerine, resulting in enhanced myocardial perfusion. Although nitroglycerine has no known teratogenic effects, it is important to control the dosage carefully to minimize maternal hypotension and fetal discomfort.

In the thrombolytic era, there has been no evidence that using nitroglycerine reduces infarct size or death. Nitroglycerine must be used with caution in patients with inferior MI and right ventricular involvement since it might induce severe hypotension.

In the treatment of AMI, β-blockers and calcium-channel blockers (risk category C) are controversial. Despite published studies on their safety during pregnancy, the cardiologist in charge of the patient should consult with the obstetrician before deciding to administer these medications.

Thrombolytic drugs are utilized as an immediate treatment for coronary artery blockage and the prevention or restriction of MI. The agents of choice include tissue plasminogen activators (t-PA), such as tenecteplase and reteplase. The risk/benefit ratio of thrombolytic medicines is controversial with bleeding, preterm childbirth, and incoordinate uterine contractions among the possible side effects. The decision to use thrombolytic drugs should be decided by the cardiologist and therefore the obstetrician in consultation.

Rescue percutaneous coronary intervention (PCI) of the infarct-related artery may be done with satisfactory outcomes in instances of MI that do not respond to thrombolytic medications.[15]

Percutaneous coronary intervention, also known as percutaneous transluminal coronary angioplasty, is a kind of percutaneous coronary angioplasty.[13] In patients with angina pectoris and AMI, percutaneous coronary intervention (PCI) for the treatment of coronary artery occlusive disease might be a well-established therapeutic option. The safety of drug-eluting stents in pregnant women is still unclear because all documented stenting during the acute phase of MI during pregnancy was done with bare metal stents.

Because drug-eluting stents necessitate long-term antiplatelet therapy, which raises the chance of C-section births in individuals with cardiovascular disease, utilizing one during pregnancy is dangerous and should be avoided if at all possible.

In one small study, coronary artery bypass was linked to a maternal death rate of 1–2% and a fetal loss rate of roughly 33%; however, the mortality rate in the pregnant population does not differ from that observed in the nonpregnant population; however, the limited available information prevents drawing definitive conclusions about the proteome. Women should be addressed if they have an acute cardiac incident during pregnancy. Cardiologists, obstetricians, obstetric anesthetists, and, when necessary, cardiothoracic surgeons worked together in a very collaborative manner. When taken in amounts <150 mg/day, aspirin is safe during pregnancy. Although there are no significant datasets demonstrating the use of clopidogrel during pregnancy, published findings do not appear to suggest fetal harm, and women should be counseled about the lack of knowledge.

LABOR AND DELIVERY: TIMING OF DELIVERY

An MI during pregnancy is a symptom that delivery should be postponed following the infarction. The time between the infarct and delivery is inversely related to maternal mortality. After an infarct, every effort should be made to stabilize the patient and postpone delivery. It is thought that the maternal cardiovascular system is unstable after an infarct, and that the stress of labor on top of that might cause rapid worsening. Within 5–7 days following the AMI, the maternal ventricular function recovers to a state of stability, lowering the risk of further labor stress.

Because of the scarcity of prospective data and the effect of individual patient's characteristics in this context, there are no defined standards for obstetric treatment. Individualized interventions must be tailored to the mother's cardiac condition and gestational age. If a danger of premature birth exists, maternal steroid injections should be given as soon as possible. Due to the increased risk of maternal death following AMI, birth should be postponed for 2–3 weeks if at all feasible.

Obstetric and maternal characteristics should be used to determine the method of birth (vaginal or elective C-section), as neither is connected to a higher death rate. Although vaginal birth is associated with a lower risk of vaginal blood loss, infection, and thrombosis, an elective C-section avoids the hemodynamic shifts of labor and allows for a rapid delivery with all members of the multidisciplinary team present.

Because a protracted labor may negatively affect myocardial workload due to larger elevations in preload from uterine contractions, the Bishop score and fetal health will decide the time of vaginal birth (spontaneous versus inducement of labor). An epidural analgesia is indicated if a vaginal birth is attempted to diminish pain-related sympathetic activity as well as the urge to push. Women must labor in the left lateral position to lessen the impact of uterine pressure on hemodynamic circulation.

Continuous maternal cardiovascular monitoring, which includes pulse oximetry and ECG, is required in addition to supplemental oxygen. Continuous fetal monitoring is also necessary.

Invasive monitoring with an arterial catheter is also recommended if left ventricular function is severely reduced or in women who have had a recent cardiac episode. To minimize the undesirable hemodynamic impact of the Valsalva technique and to shorten the labor, it is typically suggested to abbreviate the second stage with instrumental delivery.

ANALGESIA IN LABOR

With patients who have had a prior MI, epidural analgesia is the preferable technique of pain relief. The following are some of the advantages of epidural analgesia: There is a significant reduction in discomfort, stress, and anxiety, as well as a reduction in afterload, which decreases the amount of cardiac effort necessary.

Epidural anesthesia may have a known potential drawback of lowering preload. This problem can be avoided by ensuring that the patient is well hydrated at the time of epidural induction. In patients who have had a prior MI, vasopressors are contraindicated in the treatment of epidural-induced hypotension.

MODE OF DELIVERY

In patients who have had the MI, the most popular mode of delivery is vaginal delivery. C-sections should only be performed on individuals who have obstetrical reasons and should be treated with caution. Maternal mortality is reported to be 14% with vaginal birth after MI, compared to 23% with C-section delivery.

The elimination of surgical stress, the lack of a general anesthetic, a decreased incidence of postpartum infection, and less blood loss are all advantages of vaginal delivery. Patients who are born vaginally are more likely to ambulate sooner, lowering their risk of thromboembolic illness. After a vaginal birth, analgesics are typically not required. The drawbacks of vaginal delivery include the lengthening of the birth process and, as a result, the unpredictability of the delivery mode and timing.

The advantages of a C-section are that it allows for a controlled birth with all of the professionals and equipment needed to care for both the mother and the unborn on hand right once. The use of a C-section is linked to a shorter period of hemodynamic alterations throughout the delivery process. Increased blood loss, which can be linked to hypotension, which can either induce a second infarct episode or result in an expansion of the current infarct, is one of the drawbacks of C-section. C-section is also linked to a higher risk of infection, pulmonary morbidity, and metabolic demands associated with surgery and the recovery period.

Caesarean section is the preferred mode of delivery in patients who have developed acute heart failure as a result of the MI. When a patient chooses to try a vaginal birth, the second stage is generally reduced with the use of outlet forceps or a vacuum extractor.

MANAGEMENT OF THE THIRD STAGE OF LABOR

In the case of a patient who has had a simple vaginal delivery, there is no need for active intervention in the third stage. When a patient has had a difficult third stage of labor, intensive therapy is always recommended. Patients with postpartum hemorrhage, in particular, should be treated as soon as possible. In a patient who has had a prior MI, oxytocin is the medication of choice for reducing postpartum hemorrhage. Compounds containing ergot are not recommended. Prostaglandin F2a's utility and safety in patients with MI have yet to be established.[4]

INDICATION FOR INVASIVE MONITORING

Only patients with evidence of or a strong suspicion of heart failure should utilize Swan-Ganz catheters and arterial lines to monitor blood pressure, central venous pressure, pulmonary artery, and pulmonary wedge pressure.

Flowchart 1 outlines the management of AMI in pregnancy.

Flowchart 1: Management of acute myocardial infarction (MI) in pregnancy.[4]

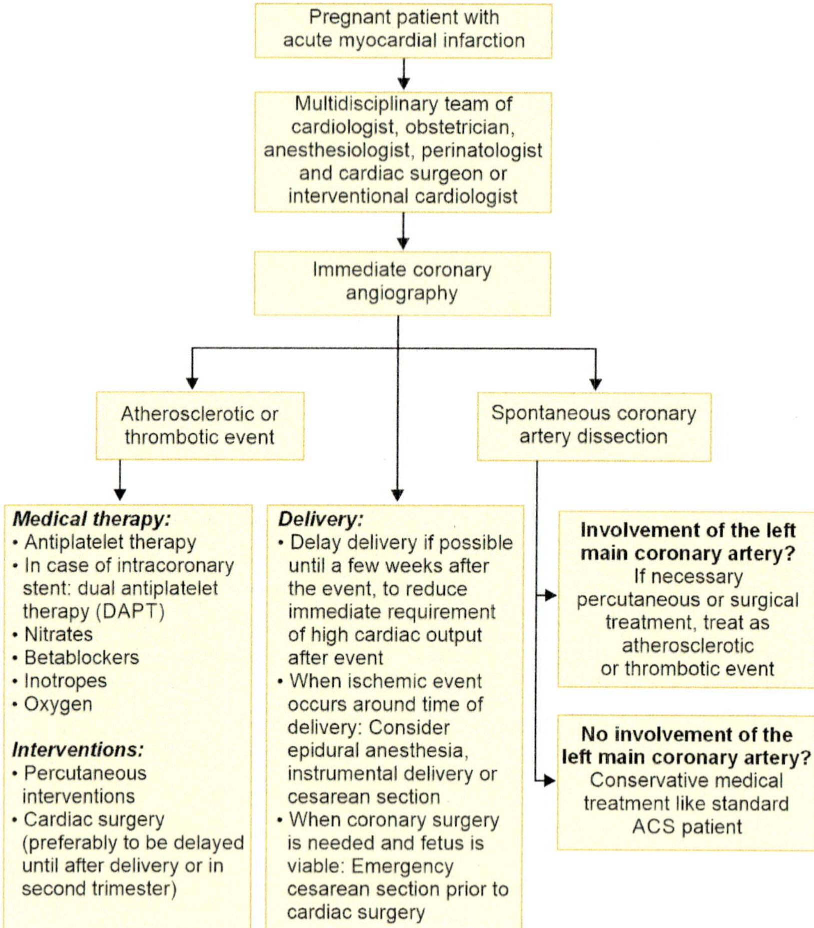

(ACS: acute coronary syndrome)

Source: Cauldwell M, Baris L, Roos-Hesselink JW, et al. Ischaemic heart disease and pregnancy. Heart. 2019;105:189-95.

CONCLUSION

The significant hemodynamic changes that accompany pregnancy can considerably exacerbate the risk of myocardial infarction (MI) in women with undiagnosed coronary artery disease (CAD). The expanded intravascular and plasma volume, elevated stroke volume, and increased cardiac output during the different trimesters collectively pose a heightened strain on the cardiovascular system. This situation necessitates a vigilant and tailored approach to diagnosing and managing ischemic heart disease during pregnancy.

The complex interplay of predisposing factors like smoking, age, and pre-existing conditions such as hypertension or hyperlipidemia, further complicates the cardiovascular risk profile during pregnancy. Moreover, the diagnostic challenge posed by pregnancy-related physiological changes underscores the need for careful interpretation of clinical presentations and judicious use of diagnostic tools that minimize risk to the fetus. The management of IHD in pregnant women requires a coordinated, multidisciplinary approach, involving obstetricians, cardiologists, and other healthcare professionals to optimize both maternal and fetal outcomes.

Through individualized patient management strategies, continuous monitoring, and appropriate therapeutic interventions, healthcare providers can mitigate the risks associated with IHD during pregnancy. Ultimately, the goal is to ensure the safety and health of both the mother and the developing fetus, guiding them through the complexities of pregnancy with the least possible complication from cardiovascular diseases.

REFERENCES

1. Kealey A. Coronary artery disease and myocardial infarction in pregnancy: a review of epidemiology, diagnosis, and medical and surgical management. Canadian j cardiol. 2010;26(6):185-9.
2. Chung WK, Austin ED, Best DH, Brown LM, Elliott CG, City SL, et al. HHS Public Access. 2015;31(307):544-7.
3. Kennedy BB, Baird SMM. Acute Myocardial Infarction in Pregnancy: An Update. J Perinat Neonatal Nurs. 2016;30(1):13-24.
4. Cauldwell M, Baris L, Roos-Hesselink JW, Johnson MR. Ischaemic heart disease and pregnancy. Heart. 2019;105(3):189-95.
5. Bondagji NS. Ischaemic heart disease in pregnancy. J Saudi Heart Assoc [Internet]. 2012;24(2):89-97.
6. Dufour P, Orazi G, Vinatier D, Tordjeman N, Theeten G, Decoulx E, et al. Myocardial infarction and pregnancy. J Gynecol Obstet Biol la Reprod. 1996;25(7):746-51.
7. Lameijer H, Burchill LJ, Baris L, Ruys TP, Roos-Hesselink JW, Mulder BJM, et al. Pregnancy in women with pre-existent ischaemic heart disease: a systematic review with individualised patient data. Heart. 2019;105(11):873-80.
8. Meads C, Cummins C, Jolly K, Stevens A, Burls A, Hyde C. Coronary artery stents in the treatment of ischaemic heart disease: a rapid and systematic review. Health Technol Assess. 2000;4(23):1-153.
9. Alatorre CI, Hoogwerf BJ, Deeg MA, Nelson DR, Hunter TM, Ng WT, et al. Factors associated with stroke, myocardial infarction, ischemic heart disease, unstable angina, or mortality in patients from real world clinical practice with newly-diagnosed type 2 diabetes and early glycemic control. Curr Med Res Opin. 2018;34(2):337-43.
10. Morris F, Brady WJ. ABC of clinical electrocardiography: Acute myocardial infarction-Part I. BMJ (Clin res ed.). 2002;324(7341):831-4.
11. Dupuganti MM, Ganga V. Acute myocardial infarction in pregnancy: Current diagnosis and management approaches. Indian Heart J. 2019;71(5):367-74.

12. Baird SM, Kennedy B. Myocardial infarction in pregnancy. J Perinat Neonatal Nurs. 2006;20(4):311-21; quiz 322-3.
13. Ismail S, Wong C, Rajan P, Vidovich MI. ST-elevation acute myocardial infarction in pregnancy: 2016 update. Clin Cardiol. 2017;40(6):399-406.
14. Smilowitz NR, Gupta N, Guo Y, Zhong J, Weinberg CR, Reynolds HR, et al. Acute Myocardial Infarction During Pregnancy and the Puerperium in the United States. Mayo Clin Proc. 2018;93(10):1404-14.
15. Gibson P, Narous M, Firoz T, Chou D, Barreix M, Say L, et al.; WHO Maternal Morbidity Working Group. Incidence of myocardial infarction in pregnancy: a systematic review and meta-analysis of population-based studies. Eur Heart J Qual Care Clin Outcomes. 2017;3(3):198-207.

10 CHAPTER

Anesthesia and Analgesia in Cardiac Diseases in Pregnancy

INTRODUCTION

Pregnancy leads to physiological changes in the cardiovascular system. The intravascular volume increases by 40–50% which peaks in second trimester. There is decrease in systemic vascular resistance (SVR) throughout pregnancy but the normal mean arterial pressure (MAP) is maintained even though the cardiac output is increased by 30–40%. There are fluctuations in cardiac output during labor and postpartum with cardiac output increasing by 40–50%. With each uterine contraction there is an autotransfusion to the central blood volume, leading to an increase in cardiac output of 10–25%.[1] Pregnancy is a hypercoagulable state, hence, there is an increased risk of thrombus formation. Another factor to consider is the hypercoagulability that comes with pregnancy, as well as the potential need for anticoagulation, particularly in individuals who are at higher risk of arterial thrombosis and embolization (prosthetic heart valve).[2]

DISEASE OF THE VALVULAR HEART

Rheumatic fever is the most prevalent cause of valvular heart disease. Univentricular or biventricular failure, atrial dysrhythmias, systemic or pulmonary embolism, and infective endocarditis are all common pregnancy problems, with an overall frequency of difficulties estimated at 15% of all valvular disease patients. Patients who are pregnant tolerate regurgitant heart disease well because their plasma volume is reduced and their SVR is reduced, resulting in higher cardiac output.[3] As the pregnancy advances, stenotic valvular disease is poorly tolerated due to the inability to increase cardiac output in relation to the increased plasma volume preload.

MITRAL STENOSIS

As left ventricular diastolic filling is prolonged, tachycardia should be avoided. Asymptomatic patients at term required strict observation only without need for invasive monitoring but patients with marked symptoms are at high risk at term and postpartum period and should be provided with continuous monitoring. In patient with fixed CO in the immediate postpartum period, there is a sudden increase in circulatory volume which is poorly tolerated.

In order to minimize hemodynamic alterations, lumbar epidural is the best method of analgesia for vaginal delivery. Analgesia is better on addition of opioids in order to dilute anesthetic mixture without increasing the chances of sympathetic blockade.

Appropriate segmental and perineal anesthesia lowers catecholamine-induced heart rate increases and the desire to push, allowing fetal descent to be completed by uterine contractions and avoiding the negative consequences of Valsalva's maneuver during the second stage of labor. When neuraxial anesthesia is not an option, the pudendal nerve can be blocked to relieve pain.

The extra risks of significant fluid shift due to anesthetic method, operational blood loss, and fluid mobilization in the postpartum period must all be considered when choosing an anesthetic for caesarean birth. The use of epidural anesthesia over spinal anesthesia is preferable because the former causes a delayed start of blockage and therefore more controlled hemodynamic changes.[1]

Prophylactic ephedrine treatment and arbitrary intravascular volume loading should be avoided in the symptomatic patient. Instead, a careful titration of anesthetic level allows for cautious and appropriate intravenous fluid supply, guided by hemodynamic monitoring. These people may be at risk for hypotension during epidural anesthesia due to venous pooling and previous β-adrenergic suppression and diuretic therapy.

Ephedrine, the most common vasopressor, should be avoided since it might cause tachycardia. Instead, low-dose phenylephrine can help to restore the mother's blood pressure while having little or no effect on uteroplacental perfusion. If sympathetic stimulation related with laryngoscopy and intubation, as well as suction and extubation, is reduced, general anesthesia may also give a highly stable hemodynamic course. Anesthetics and/or β-adrenergic inhibition may be used to achieve this.[4] The use of medications that often cause tachycardia should be avoided while inducing general anesthesia. Opioids, neuromuscular blocking medications, nitrous oxide, and oxygen are used to maintain anesthesia. To avoid tachycardia, the emergence must be carefully managed.

AORTIC STENOSIS

Because the natural history of this lesion forming as a result of rheumatic heart disease often takes three to four decades to reach a severity adequate to generate symptoms, aortic stenosis seldom causes pregnancy difficulties. On the other hand, women with congenital bicuspid aortic valves and those who have had bacterial endocarditis may develop significant aortic stenosis during pregnancy. Severe aortic stenosis is defined as a narrowing of the valve area to $<1\ cm^2$ and a transvalvular gradient of 50 mm Hg, resulting in a substantial increase in valvular afterload to left ventricular ejection.

Although contractility is occasionally retained, the left ventricle hypertrophies properly and concentrically and becomes significantly less compliant. Because of the increased blood volume and decreased SVR, the transvalvular gradient rises gradually throughout pregnancy. The following objectives are included in anesthesia management:[5]

- Avoiding tachycardia and bradycardia
- Preserving appropriate preload in the left ventricle so that it can generate adequate cardiac output across the stenotic valve
- Keeping hemodynamic parameters within a small therapeutic window.

Invasive monitoring with peripheral and pulmonary artery catheters is recommended for patients with transvalvular gradients higher than 50 mm Hg and symptomatic aortic stenosis. The use of segmental epidural anesthesia for labor analgesia is contentious because these individuals may not be able to endure the reductions in preload and afterload caused by sympathetic blocking. Other options include subarachnoid or epidural opioids, either alone or in combination with an epidural segmental anesthetic.[6] The circulatory effects of spinal opioids are negligible; cardiac contractility is unaffected; preload is maintained; and most importantly, SVR is not reduced.

Either properly titrated epidural anesthesia or general anesthesia can be used during caesarean (C)-section. Myocardial depression caused by volatile anesthetics should be avoided under general anesthesia, just as it should be avoided in a parturient with mitral stenosis.

MITRAL INSUFFICIENCY

The second most common valvular lesion in pregnancy is mitral valve insufficiency and regurgitation. Most people with mitral regurgitation handle pregnancy well because chronic left ventricular volume overload and work are typically well tolerated, with symptoms appearing later in life after reproductive age. Atrial fibrillation, bacterial endocarditis needing antibiotic prophylaxis, systemic embolization, and pulmonary congestion are all possible complications during pregnancy. Mitral regurgitation is considerably less frequent in pregnant women than congenital mitral valve prolapses, which occurs in 10–17% of pregnancies.[7] Mitral regurgitation is a well-tolerated and largely harmless condition. Regurgitation caused by an inadequate mitral valve causes persistent volume overload and dilatation of the left ventricle as a result of the pathophysiology. The increase in plasma volume with pregnancy progression may cause pulmonary venous congestion if left ventricular impairment has been present for a long time and is severe. The decreased SVR associated with pregnancy, on the other hand, may help to enhance forward flow across the aortic valve at the expense of regurgitant flow. Increases in SVR as a result of labor discomfort, uterine contractions, or surgical stimulation may result in an increase in regurgitant blood flow, which may result in abrupt left ventricular failure.[8] Appropriate labor analgesia should reduce peripheral vasoconstriction, reducing the rise in left ventricular afterload associated with labor discomfort. Sympathetic blockade reduces SVR and is beneficial in this situation; the caveat is that venous capacitance increases, thus preload must be increased gradually to preserve left ventricular filling capacity. At term, asymptomatic patients are unlikely to need invasive observation. Invasive monitoring should be performed in symptomatic patients.

AORTIC INSUFFICIENCY

Congenital aortic insufficiency is typically linked with various disorders; however, acquired aortic insufficiency can be caused by rheumatic heart disease or endocarditis in conjunction with aortic root dissection. Because rheumatic fever symptoms usually appear in the fourth or fifth decade of life, the majority of women who have this as their primary lesion have easy pregnancies. Chronic left ventricular volume overload is the underlying pathology, resulting in hypertrophy and dilation, as well as increased compliance. While myocardial oxygen requirements are increased due to hypertrophy, a decrease in diastolic pressure and an increase in left ventricular end-diastolic pressure may result in a decrease in perfusion pressure and therefore oxygen delivery. As a result, anesthetic concerns center on minimizing pain and, as a result, catecholamine-induced increases in SVR thus avoiding bradycardia, which helps to prolong the time for regurgitant flow and avoiding myocardial depressants, which may exacerbate failure.[9] The anesthetic issues are similar to those encountered in patients with mitral regurgitation, and epidural anesthesia is favored during labor and delivery to avoid peripheral vasoconstriction. Any patient exhibiting symptoms of congestive heart failure should be monitored invasively. Complications such as thromboembolism, valvular outflow obstruction, endocarditis, and hemolysis can occur in parturient who have had their mitral or aortic valves replaced. To avoid thromboembolic consequences, anticoagulation with coumarin derivatives is typically required. To minimize congenital abnormalities in the fetus, heparin is typically used instead of coumarin anticoagulants during pregnancy. Anticoagulation increases the risk of an epidural-spinal hematoma and makes regional anesthesia impossible to employ. When regional anesthetic was used low-molecular weight heparin (enoxaparin) was linked to spinal epidural hematoma. This is most likely owing to the fact that it has a longer half-life than unfractionated heparin. As a result, it is recommended that regional anesthetic not be used until the medicine has been taken off the market for at least 12–24 hours, depending on the dosage.[9,10]

Continuing heparinization throughout labor and delivery, as well as using systemic analgesia for labor and general anesthetic for delivery, is one option. Another option with unfractionated heparin is to stop taking it right before labor and delivery, correct the coagulation levels, utilize regional anesthetic, and then start taking it again 12 hours later.[11]

CONGENITAL HEART DISEASE

Congenital heart disease is the most prevalent cause of cardiac issues in pregnant patients. With the introduction of palliative surgery or comprehensive repair of congenital abnormalities, patients are more likely to live to reproductive age. The pregnancy and birth of many of these individuals are likely to be uncomplicated.

LEFT-TO-RIGHT SHUNTS

In adults with congenital heart disease, a ventricular septal defect (VSD) occurs in 7% of cases. In the absence of pulmonary hypertension, patients with untreated lesions perform well throughout pregnancy. Maternal mortality varies from 7 to 40% in the limited number of individuals with big VSDs and concomitant pulmonary hypertension. Severe right ventricular failure with shunt reversal (Eisenmenger's syndrome) is the most common consequence. By increasing the left-to-right shunt, increases in plasma volume, cardiac output, and heart rate during pregnancy may worsen pulmonary hypertension. The primary peripartum treatment objectives are founded on the recognition that significant increases in peripheral vascular resistance and heart rate may be poorly tolerated, with ventricular failure being a clear possibility. Shunt reversal and hypoxia can result from sudden increases in pulmonary vascular resistance (PVR) and right ventricular dysfunction.[12]

Segmental epidural anesthesia using local anesthetics, opioids, or a mix of the two is ideal for labor and vaginal delivery. C-section anesthesia can be achieved with either a slow titration of an epidural anesthetic agent to allow time for pressure changes to be corrected, or with a general anesthetic agent that combines opioid and inhalation techniques to depress the adrenergic response to tracheal intubation and minimize myocardial depression.

Despite the fact that all popular types of labor analgesia are effective, lumbar epidural analgesia during labor, vaginal birth, or C-section reduces the risks of higher SVR. As long as rises in SVR are avoided and sinus rhythm is maintained, general anesthesia during C-section is generally tolerated.[13] Avoiding increases in SVR and hypervolemia are two important anesthetic concerns. In individuals with preexisting pulmonary hypertension and right ventricular impairment, however, abrupt reductions in SVR may result in shunt reversal. Continuous lumbar epidural analgesia for labor reduces the pain-related rise in SVR. If increases in SVR due to tracheal intubation and surgical stimulation are properly controlled, epidural or general anesthesia is suitable for a C-section.

RIGHT-TO-LEFT SHUNTS

Pneumotension, a right-to-left intracardiac shunt (due to pulmonary hypertension superimposed over a previously left-to-right shunt), and arterial hypoxemia make up Eisenmenger's syndrome. Patients with this disease do not handle pregnancy well. The maternal mortality rate is believed to be between 30 and 50%. In individuals with congenital cardiac disease, this entity is responsible for around half of the maternal mortality. The main focus of anesthetic considerations is to avoid any reduction in SVR or cardiac depression. Hypotension caused by a variety of factors, including conduction block or bleeding, can lead to inadequate right ventricular pressures to perfuse the hypertensive pulmonary arterial bed, resulting in rapid death. If SVR is maintained, analgesia during vaginal birth can be provided using systemic opioids, subarachnoid opioids, or the judicious administration of a segmental epidural. The use of only an epidural or a subarachnoid opioid during the first stage of labor has been proposed as the safest option. A caudal epidural block may be preferred to a lumbar epidural block for the second stage of labor because dense perineal analgesia can be delivered without significant sympathetic blocking. Although regional anesthesia for elective caesarean birth has been recorded, general anesthesia is the safest way to deliver via C-section.

The postpartum period, regardless of the anesthetic method used, is arguably the most probable time for life-threatening hypoxemia, cardiac dysrhythmias, and thromboembolic events to occur; in fact, most maternal fatalities occur in the first postpartum week.

Primary pulmonary hypertension is more common in women of reproductive age, and it is linked to a high maternal death rate (>50%). During childbirth and the puerperium, the majority of fatalities occur. The severity of the condition affects the signs and symptoms, which are produced by a fixed low cardiac output, pulmonary hypertension, and right ventricular compromise.[14]

The focus of anesthetic considerations is on determining the severity of the disease and its response to treatment, maintaining hemodynamic stability, and delivering the appropriate analgesia and anesthesia for labor and delivery. Underventilation, pharmacological drugs, lung hyperinflation, and stress all enhance PVR, therefore, the anesthesiologist must first consider this when choosing an anesthetic regimen. Furthermore, right ventricular volume reductions caused by intravascular volume depletion, venodilation, or aortocaval compression are poorly tolerated.

Reduced SVR as a result of sympathetic blockade or volatile anesthetics may result in substantial decompensation, as the circulatory system may be unable to cope with the decreased afterload. Finally, right ventricular contractility may be minimal, and the addition of negative inotropic anesthetics may result in significant cardiac function decline. Throughout labor and the postpartum period, the parturient should be monitored using an ECG, pulse oximetry, radial artery catheter, and pulmonary artery catheter.

Systemic opioid analgesics with pudendal nerve block may be the best way to manage labor and vaginal delivery. Only if the block is gradually titrated in a restricted dermatomal manner from T10 to L1 may epidural analgesia with a local anesthetic be delivered. First-stage analgesia can also be achieved using subarachnoid or epidural opioids. A caudal or pudendal block might be used to help with vaginal birth. Regional anesthesia is best avoided with C-section deliveries, and a gradual induction with either high-dose opioids or an inhaled medication is indicated. This is required to avoid substantial PVR elevations during laryngoscopy. Uterine stimulants should probably be avoided since they have been linked to substantial increases in PVR.[7,10.]

CORONARY ARTERY DISEASE

With a reported prevalence of 1 in 10,000 births, coronary artery disease is uncommon in women of reproductive age. Only 13% of pregnant women who had a myocardial infarction (MI) had a known history of coronary artery disease, according to one study; total maternal mortality was 37%, rising to 45% if the MI occurred in the third trimester. General treatment guidelines presently include interventions such as bed rest, nitrate therapy for preload reduction, and conduction anesthetic during delivery to reduce heart workload. β-blockers and nitrates, for example, should be taken throughout the pregnancy, labor, delivery, and puerperium.

Although systemic opioid analgesia can provide adequate pain relief, continuous regional anesthetic for labor and delivery should be started as soon as possible. Reduced preload and afterload, as well as reduced myocardial effort, are all beneficial benefits of regional anesthetic. Because coronary artery perfusion is dependent on diastolic pressure, significant and abrupt reductions in afterload must be avoided. Significant reductions in SVR can also trigger reflex tachycardia, which can raise cardiac workload enough to cause ischemia. In the unanesthetized parturient, epidural anesthesia effectively reduces the gradual increases in central venous pressure and cardiac output that occur throughout labor. To minimize tachycardia, it is recommended that epinephrine should be left out of the test dosage and then the block should be created using slower-acting local anesthetics such as bupivacaine or ropivacaine. In addition, it has been suggested that a dilute local anesthetic solution should be supplemented with an epidural opioid.

According to the patient's baseline ejection fraction and hemodynamic response to contractions, fetal descent during the second stage of labor should be by force of uterine contraction, with Valsalva's maneuver (which rapidly reduces preload) avoided. A mild spinal anesthetic (saddle block) gives good circumstances for an aided birth when epidural analgesia is not used for the first stage of labor.[1] A gradually titrated dose of epidural anesthetic can be used to successfully conduct an elective C-section, allowing for cautious intravenous fluid infusion to preserve pulmonary capillary wedge pressure and blood pressure. Given the fast onset of sympathetic block, which has a high risk of hypotension and reflex tachycardia, spinal anesthesia is significantly less desirable. The anesthesiologist must consider the significance of reducing the cardiovascular reaction to the stress of tracheal intubation and surgery while providing general anesthesia for the C-section.

Regional anesthesia is best avoided with C-section deliveries, and a gradual induction with either high-dose opioids or an inhaled medication is indicated. This is required to avoid substantial PVR elevations during laryngoscopy.

IDIOPATHIC HYPERTROPHIC SUBAORTIC STENOSIS

Idiopathic hypertrophic subaortic stenosis (IHSS) is a disease with no known cause, although it appears to be inherited as an autosomal dominant characteristic in at least one-third of the individuals. Marked hypertrophy of the left ventricle and interventricular septum, as well as blockage of the left ventricular outflow pathway during systole by the hypertrophied muscle, are the major characteristics of this cardiomyopathy. The disease often manifests in the second to fourth decades of life. Angina pectoris, dizziness, and exertional dyspnea are also common symptoms. Left ventricular hypertrophy, a systolic ejection murmur, and a third heart sound are all physical findings. An ECG will reveal left ventricular hypertrophy, as well as signs of Wolff–Parkinson–White syndrome and aberrant Q waves in certain instances.

The left ventricle's volume during systole, the force of left ventricular contraction, and the degree of left ventricular distention during systole all have an effect on the degree of blockage. To maintain a full left ventricle, the patient needs a high preload, a low-contractile force to keep the outflow route as narrow as possible, and a high SVR to maintain a swollen left ventricle during systole. The use of β-adrenergic blocking medications to decrease myocardial contractility and heart rate is the mainstay of treatment. Hypovolemia, reduced SVR, and increases in cardiac contractility are not well tolerated by patients with IHSS. Pregnancy's circulatory and hemodynamic alterations affect people with IHSS in different ways, depending on the degree and type of the condition.[15]

Because it increases preload, the increase in blood volume associated with pregnancy should have a positive impact. The often-seen rise in heart rate and stroke volume during pregnancy can be harmful, and the reduction in SVR, which occurs in the second trimester, can also be harmful to cardiac function. The therapeutic aims during parturition should be to minimize pain-related increases in catecholamine levels, to maintain preload with enough intravenous fluid supply, and to avoid Valsalva's maneuver, which abruptly decreases preload.

Monitoring with an arterial line and a pulmonary artery catheter will provide the necessary data for optimal treatment. Systemic opioids, inhalation analgesics, or paracervical block have all been recommended for analgesia during the first stage of labor. Because of the possibility for both venodilation and arterial dilatation, resulting in reduced SVR, regional analgesia has been thoroughly thought-out to be a significant danger. However, if cautious progressive titration of continuous lumbar epidural analgesia is performed, this may be avoided. From T10 to L2, a low dose offers sufficient analgesia with little sympathetic blockage, retaining preload. Analgesia is best achieved by diluting a local anesthetic agent and adding an opioid, such as fentanyl. Subarachnoid opioids may also be administered, removing the possibility of sympathetic blocking.

A patient with IHSS was effectively treated with a combination of spinal and epidural analgesics. Pudendal block, appropriately prolonged epidural analgesia, or saddle block are all options for vaginal birth. The saddle block obliterates the bulk of sympathetic nerve components by involving the spinal segments L2 to S5. If hypotension necessitates the use of a vasopressor, ephedrine should be avoided since it induces tachycardia and increased cardiac contractility. To reduce the effect on the uterine arteries, a pure vasoconstricting medication like phenylephrine should be used in the lowest effective dosage. Phenylephrine is the primary vasopressor for treating hypotension in these individuals in many centers.

Anesthesia for caesarean birth comes with its own set of difficulties. Because of the increased blood loss, the left uterine displacement must be maintained, and volume requirements must be carefully monitored. It will be necessary to conduct invasive monitoring. For the reasons stated above, regional anesthesia is typically avoided, and the amount of anesthetic necessary is plainly likely to cause significant sympathetic blocking, which has unfavorable implications.[2,15] Nonetheless, a carefully titrated epidural anesthetic with continuous compensation for the resulting hemodynamic alterations could be sufficient. Many people choose general anesthesia, despite the fact that the best approach has yet to be discovered and experience is limited. Oxytocin should be used with caution since it has a tendency to lower SVR and induce tachycardia when given too quickly. **Flowchart 1** shows the management algorithm for an obstetric patient with inadequate neuraxial anesthesia.

Flowchart 1: Management algorithm for an obstetric patient with inadequate neuraxial anesthesia.

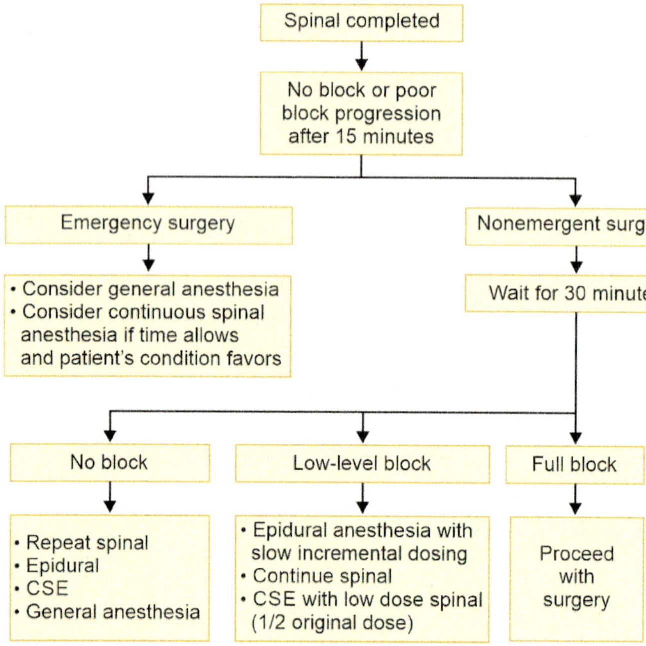

(CSE: combined spinal–epidural)

CONCLUSION

Pregnancy induces profound physiological changes within the cardiovascular system, adapting to the increased demands of both mother and fetus. These changes include a significant rise in intravascular volume, up to 50% by the second trimester, and an elevation in cardiac output by 30-40% to accommodate this volume. Systemic vascular resistance (SVR) consistently decreases, yet mean arterial pressure (MAP) remains stable due to compensatory mechanisms. Labor and the postpartum period further alter cardiac output, particularly during uterine contractions, creating temporary autotransfusions that increase central blood volume.

Moreover, pregnancy poses an increased thrombotic risk due to its inherently hypercoagulable state, necessitating vigilant monitoring and potential anticoagulation in high-risk cases. Valvular heart disease, particularly when stenotic, presents unique challenges, as the cardiovascular system's limited capacity to increase output can lead to decompensation. Managing such conditions during pregnancy requires a nuanced understanding of these physiological changes and a careful balance in the delivery of anesthesia and analgesia to minimize risk and stabilize hemodynamics.

The choice of analgesic and anesthetic techniques during labor and delivery must consider these physiological alterations to optimize maternal and fetal outcomes. Tailored approach ensures that the cardiovascular demands of pregnancy and delivery are met with minimal risk, highlighting the intricate balance required in the management of cardiac diseases in pregnancy.

REFERENCES

1. Arendt KW, Lindley KJ. Obstetric anesthesia management of the patient with cardiac disease. Int J Obstet Anesth [Internet]. 2019;37(September 2018):73-85.
2. Kuczkowski KM. Labor analgesia for the parturient with lumbar tattoos: What does an obstetrician need to know? Arch Gynecol Obstet. 2006;274(5):310-2.
3. Luthra A, Bajaj R, Jafra A, Jangra K, Arya VK. Anesthesia in pregnancy with heart disease. Saudi J Anaesth. 2017;11(4):454-71.
4. Hink E, Luitjes SH, Bolte AC. PP150. Pregnancy outcome in women with heart disease in a single tertiary care center. Pregnancy Hypertens. 2012;2(3):320.
5. Habib AS. What's new in obstetric anesthesia in 2017? Int J Obstet Anesth. 2019;38:119-26.
6. Meng ML, Arendt KW. Obstetric Anesthesia and Heart Disease: Practical Clinical Considerations. Anesthesiology. 2021;135(1):164-83.
7. Shatalin D, Jaber M, Barsky D, Avitan T, Grisaru-Granovsky S, Gozal Y, et al. Outcome of Peripartum Anesthesia in Women with Valvular Disease. Rom J Anaesth Intensive Care. 2020;27(1):11-4.
8. Warrick CM, Hart JE, Lynch AM, Hawkins JA, Bucklin BA. Prevalence and descriptive analysis of congenital heart disease in parturients: obstetric, neonatal, and anesthetic outcomes. J Clin Anesth. 2015;27(6):492-8.
9. Mignon A. Conséquences foetales des techniques d'anesthésie au cours du travail [Effects of maternal analgesia and anesthesia on the fetus and the newborn]. J Gynecol Obstet Biol Reprod (Paris). 2008;37(Suppl 1):S46-55.
10. Ranasinghe JS. Complete heart block in pregnancy: case report, analysis, and review of anesthetic management. J Clin Anesth. 2016;33:58-61.
11. Mace HS, Paech MJ, McDonnell NJ. Obesity and obstetric anaesthesia. Anaesth Intensive Care. 2011;39(4):559-70.
12. Turnbull J, Bell R. Obstetric anaesthesia and peripartum management. Best Pract Res Clin Obstet Gynaecol. 2014;28(4):593-605.
13. Levin H, LaSala A. Intrapartum obstetric management. Semin Perinatol. 2014;38(5):245-51.
14. Turker G, Gurbet A, Aksu HA. Continuous spinal analgesia in parturients with severe heart disease. Int J Obstet Anesth. 2007;16(3):297-9.
15. Kuczkowski KM. Labor analgesia for the parturient with cardiac disease: what does an obstetrician need to know? Acta Obstet Gynecol Scand. 2004;83(3):223-33.

11

CHAPTER

Contraception in Pregnancy in Heart Disease

INTRODUCTION

The importance of effective contraception in women with cardiac disease is very important. Circulatory changes in pregnancy can cause unmasking and decompensation of preexisting cardiac. Contraceptive counseling is necessary to prevent serious consequences, especially in the World Health Organization (WHO) class IV diseases.[1] **Table 1** mentions the risk of thrombosis and infection, as well as the percentage of women who will have an unexpected pregnancy during the first year of using a certain contraceptive technique.

NATURAL METHODS

There are a variety of treatments that leverage our knowledge of when conception happens in the cycle to try to avoid pregnancy. These procedures are not particularly dependable, and their effectiveness is highly dependent on how precisely they are used. They have no side effects, but if you truly want to avoid getting pregnant, these procedures are not for you.

INTRAUTERINE CONTRACEPTIVE DEVICE

Coils [intrauterine contraceptive devices (IUCDs)] are far more effective, with only one woman in every 100 becoming pregnant over the course of 5 years. There are two types: copper-wrapped and progesterone-like hormone-containing. The Mirena coil is safer to use in women who have never had children because it causes less bleeding (periods frequently stop completely) and infection than copper coils (whose wombs are more at risk of infection). After the coil is put, about 1 in 1,000 women experience a fainting episode. If no specialized help is available at the time, this might be dangerous for women who have major heart problems. If a coil is to be used, it should be placed in a hospital setting with cardiac anesthesia specialists on standby in case this rare problem occurs (an actual anesthetic is not usually necessary).[2] Ectopic pregnancy (pregnancy in the fallopian tube) is a rare but serious condition that necessitates surgical removal of all coils. The Mirena coil, on the other hand, has a very low chance of causing pregnancy (even lower than after sterilization). Mirena coils can last up to 5 years before they need to be replaced.

TABLE 1: The risk of thrombosis and infection, as well as the percentage of women who will have an unexpected pregnancy during the first year of using a certain contraceptive technique.[2]

Group	*Contraceptive type*	*Failure (typical, %)*	*Failure (optimal, %)*	*Continued use at 1 year (%)*	*Thrombosis risk*	*Infection risk*
• Highly effective (<1%) • Reversible	• Implant • IUCD	0.05 0.2 (LNG) 0.8 (copper)	0.05 0.2 0.6	84 80 78	• May be slightly increased risk • No increased risk	• Minimal • Transient bacteremia at insertion, increased PID
• Highly effective (<1%) • Irreversible	• Vasectomy • Tubal occlusion	0.15 0.5 (abdominal laparoscopic, or hysteroscopic)	0.1 0.5	100 100	• No increased risk • No increased risk	• Postoperative • Postoperative
Moderately effective (3–12%)	Injectable	• Depo-Provera 3% • Combined injectable 3%	• Depo-Provera 0.3% • Combined injectable 0.05%	56	• Depo-Provera: increased risk • Combined injectable: increased risk	Minimal, but no protection from PID
	Combined oral contraceptive	8	0.3	68	Increased risk	Minimal, but no protection from PID
	Desogestrel containing progesterone-only pill	8	0.3		No increased risk	Minimal, but no protection from PID
	Patch	8	0.3	68	Increased risk	Minimal, but no protection from PID
	Ring	8	0.3	68	Increased risk	Minimal, but no

Contd...

Contd...

Group	*Contraceptive type*	*Failure (typical, %)*	*Failure (optimal, %)*	*Continued use at 1 year (%)*	*Thrombosis risk*	*Infection risk*
Poorly effective (18–28%)	Male Condom	15	2	53	No increased risk	Reduced PID
	Diaphragm	16	6	57	No increased risk	Reduced PID
	Female Condom	21	5	49	No increased risk	Reduced PID
	Sponge	16–32 (nulliparous vs. parous)	9–20 (nulliparous vs. parous)	46–57 (parous vs. nulliparous)	No increased risk	No protection from PID
	Safe Period	25	3–5	51	No increased risk	No protection from PID
	Withdrawal	27	4	43	No increased risk	No protection from PID
	Spermicide	29	18	42	No increased risk	No protection from PID
No contraception		85	85			

(IUCD: intrauterine contraceptive device; LNG: levonorgestrel; PID: pelvic inflammatory disease)

ORAL CONTRACEPTIVE PILLS

There are two forms of oral contraceptives; those that include both estrogen and progestogen hormones (combined tablets) and those that only contain a little quantity of progestogen (low-dose pills) (the low-dose or mini-pill). The combination pill is arguably the most effective when used properly, with annual failure rates of <1 in 300 women. It offers a variety of benefits, one of which is the ability to determine the length of the time.[3] In addition, the combination tablet is available as a vaginal ring or patch. The risk of blood clotting or thrombosis is the most dangerous side effect of the combo tablet (three- to four-fold increased risk). Thrombosis affects about one in every 5,000 women each year. A small percentage of blood clots are fatal. This risk is still less than half that of dying while pregnant for the average woman. The normal low-dose or progestogen-only tablet, on the other hand, has virtually no side effects and does not cause thrombosis. On the other hand, it has a higher failure rate than the combination pill. A missed pill has a lesser risk of resulting in pregnancy since the woman has a greater window of time to remember to take her pill. These are progestogen intramuscular injections that last for 12 weeks.

Progestogen implant is a tiny implant placed beneath the skin of the upper arm. It continuously administers the hormone etonogestrel. Implanon is one of the most effective and safe contraceptive techniques available today. The implant is expected to last approximately three years. Each year, the likelihood of becoming pregnant is exceedingly low, i.e., less than one in a thousand. Nexplanon has taken the place of Implanon, which might be difficult to inject properly at times.[4]

STERILIZATION

Although very successful, sterilization is not the most effective method of contraception. When performed laparoscopically with Filshie clips, it has a 10-year failure rate of 2–3/1,000. The risk of failing throughout a lifetime is estimated to be 0.5%. When conducted at the same time as a caesarean section, the 10-year failure rate is higher (0.75%). In the failures, there is a higher risk of ectopic pregnancies, which can burst and cause severe bleeding and pain. Bilateral salpingectomy is a more reliable and permanent technique of contraception. General anesthesia is frequently used for laparoscopic sterilization. Instrumentation of the cervix can cause a vasovagal response, which may be too much for people with pulmonary vascular disease to handle. A carbon dioxide (CO_2) pneumoperitoneum is formed, reducing venous return and allowing CO_2 to be absorbed systemically. In women with right-to-left shunts, this can result in paradoxical emboli. Some of these issues can be addressed with regional anesthetic and a lower CO_2 level, but this needs trained operators.[5] A mini-laparotomy can also be performed under regional anesthesia. Sterilization is supposed to be permanent, but it can be reversed in some circumstances, thus there may be sorrow afterward. General anesthesia is frequently used for laparoscopic sterilization. A vasovagal response can occur when the cervix is instrumented, which might be dangerous. Essure is a sterilization treatment that involves hysteroscopically inserting intratubal stents into the proximal region of the fallopian tube under oral analgesia or anesthesia. 3 months later, tubal occlusion occurs due to mechanical blockage and inflammation, resulting in fibrosis. The insertion of the hysteroscope is associated with 1.85% of vasovagal episodes.[6]

Male Sterilization

Vasectomy is more effective than female sterilization, because it poses no risk to the woman. It is done under local anesthesia, although it should be a carefully examined option if used as contraceptive in the spouse of a woman with a serious medical condition. Her lifespan may be severely shortened, and he may choose to father children with a new spouse in the future.

EMERGENCY CONTRACEPTION

Within 72 hours of unprotected sexual intercourse (UPSI), women who failed to take necessary precautions against pregnancy can utilize levonorgestrel or the combined estrogen-progestogen (Yuzpe) regimen (UPSI). Due to its high annual failure rate, this is not designed to be used as a regular means of contraception.[3] They can have a copper intrauterine device (IUD) implanted within 5 days of UPSI. Levonorgestrel is a progestogen that is more well tolerated and effective than the Yuzpe combination. There are no medical reasons why it should not be used. If taken within 72 hours of UPSI, it has a 1% failure chance. Nausea (14%) and vomiting (14%) are the most common adverse effects (1%). An interaction between warfarin and levonorgestrel has been observed, resulting in a fourfold rise in the international normalized ratio (INR). In warfarin-treated patients, the Yuzpe regimen may be more suited. Copper IUDs are the best option for women who take liver enzyme inducers.[7]

PRECONCEPTION COUNSELING, RISK ASSESSMENT, AND MANAGEMENT PLANNING

Pregnancy triples or quadruples the risk of acute myocardial infarction, with the risk being 30 times greater in women over 40 years than in women under 20 years. Chronic hypertension, preeclampsia, diabetes, smoking, obesity, and hyperlipidemia are all risk factors. A myocardial infarction during pregnancy can kill up to 1 in every 13 women. Unfortunately, many of these risk factors are becoming more prevalent, and the majority of women who are afflicted are asymptomatic prior to pregnancy and have no history of heart disease. A high index of suspicion for myocardial infarction in any pregnant woman presenting with chest discomfort is thus a critical component of effective treatment. Aortic stenosis is a possibility. It is also worth thinking about dissection. If the discomfort is still severe, all pregnant women with chest pain should have an electrocardiogram (ECG) read by someone who is experienced in recognizing indications of myocardial ischemia and infarction, as well as a computed tomography or magnetic resonance imaging scan of the chest. A serum troponin I test may also be beneficial.[7]

PERIPARTUM CARDIOMYOPATHY

In the majority of instances, the etiology of peripartum cardiomyopathy is unknown. It generally appears late in pregnancy or early in the puerperium; however, it can happen up to 6 months after birth. Any pregnant or puerperal woman who complains of increased shortness of breath, especially when lying flat or at night, should be evaluated for peripartum cardiomyopathy.[8] It is easy to confuse it with preeclampsia because 25% of those affected are hypertensive.[9] An ECG, a chest X-ray, and an echocardiography should be performed on all such women.

RHEUMATIC HEART DISEASE

Many of these women may have never been screened for valvular heart disease, and others may be unaware they have it. This emphasizes the importance of a thorough cardiovascular assessment at the start of pregnancy for all women who were not born in a country with excellent medical screening in childhood, including heart auscultation.[10] Mitral valve stenosis (the most frequent lesion and the most dangerous) is a challenging clinical diagnosis, and the threshold for echocardiography should be low.

AORTIC DISSECTION

Most deaths from aortic dissection were caused by systolic hypertension, highlighting the importance of blood pressure monitoring during pregnancy and timely antihypertensive therapy if blood pressure rises. The most common major complication of Marfan syndrome is aortic dissection (which can be detected with a computed tomography scan).[11]

CONGENITAL HEART DISEASE

Despite the fact that deaths from congenital heart disease are infrequent, this problem affects roughly 0.8% of pregnant women.[12] Congenital heart disease is one of the most frequent congenital anomalies, and the majority of those who are born with it will live to adulthood, thanks to the development of successful corrective/palliative surgery in the previous 30 years.

PULMONARY HYPERTENSION

Progesterone-only contraceptives (oral daily), implant and depot-medroxy-progesterone acetate (DMPA) (every 3 months) is a better method of contraception as it avoids the harmful effects of combined oral contraceptive pills (OCPs) like the prothrombotic effect.[13] The advantage of implants is that it eliminates the need for daily medication or 3-monthly injections. These drugs can be used in patients who have been prescribed warfarin, albeit intramuscular injections should be avoided. The progesterone-only tiny pill is not suggested due to reliability issues.[14] In women who have heavy periods, the Mirena intrauterine system is incredibly successful and beneficial. The risk of vasovagal episodes, which can be fatal in PH, necessitates the use of these devices in a hospital setting.

Because the endothelin receptor blocker bosentan (but not ambrisentan) is an enzyme inducer, patients on bosentan must increase their dose, even though emergency hormonal contraception is safe for unprotected intercourse.[2]

CONCLUSION

Contraception is a complicated, at times befuddling topic that involves a slew of ethical, moral, and physical issues. Early contraception counseling is recommended, with the approach chosen based on the impact of (an undesired) pregnancy, the contraceptive method's risks and advantages, and the individual's preferences. In complicated cases, both a cardiologist and an obstetrician will be consulted, and due to a paucity of high-quality studies, the decision is almost always based on professional opinion. Progestogen-only long-acting reversible contraceptives are an appealing alternative for people with cardiovascular disease in many settings due to their ease of use and efficacy.

REFERENCES

1. Thorne S, MacGregor A, Nelson-Piercy C. Risks of contraception and pregnancy in heart disease. Heart. 2006;92(10):1520-5.
2. Roos-Hesselink JW, Cornette J, Sliwa K, Pieper PG, Veldtman GR, Johnson MR. Contraception and cardiovascular disease. Eur Heart J. 2015;36(27):1728-34.
3. Bonassi Machado R, Gandolpho AC, Santana N, Bocardo RC, Palandri N, Morassutti Machado R. Contraception for women with heart disease: an update. Minerva Ginecol. 2017;69(3):259-68.
4. Thorne S, Nelson-Piercy C, MacGregor A, Gibbs S, Crowhurst J, Panay N, et al. Pregnancy and contraception in heart disease and pulmonary arterial hypertension. J Fam Plann Reprod Health Care. 2006;32(2):75-81.
5. Head CE, Thorne SA. Congenital heart disease in pregnancy. Postgrad Med J. 2005;81(955):292-8.
6. Shum KK, Gupta T, Canobbio MM, Durst J, Shah SB. Family Planning and Pregnancy Management in Adults with Congenital Heart Disease. Prog Cardiovasc Dis. 2018;61(3-4):336-46.
7. Petrie MC, Hilfiker-Kleiner D, Mbakwem A, Hamdan R, Jackson AM, Forsyth P, et al. Pathophysiology, diagnosis and management of peripartum cardiomyopathy: a position statement from the Heart Failure Association of the

European Society of Cardiology Study Group on peripartum cardiomyopathy. Eur J Heart Fail. 2019;21(7):827-43.

8. Vigl M, Kaemmerer M, Seifert-Klauss V, Niggemeyer E, Nagdyman N, Trigas V, et al. Contraception in women with congenital heart disease. Am J Cardiol. 2010;106(9):1317-21.
9. van der Meer P, Mbakwem A, Bauersachs J. Long-term prognosis, subsequent pregnancy, contraception and overall management of peripartum cardiomyopathy: practical guidance paper from the Heart Failure Association of the European Society of Cardiology Study Group on Peripartum Cardiomyopathy. Eur J Heart Fail. 2018;20(6):951-62.
10. Lindley KJ, Madden T, Cahill AG, Ludbrook PA, Billadello JJ. Contraceptive use and unintended pregnancy in women with congenital heart disease. Obstet Gynecol. 2015;126(2):363-9.
11. Pundi KN, Pundi K, Johnson JN, Dearani JA, Bonnichsen CR, Phillips SD, et al. Contraception practices and pregnancy outcome in patients after Fontan operation. Congenit Heart Dis. 2016;11(1):63-70.
12. Ossola MW, Duiella SF, Zaina B, Fedele L. Congenital heart disease: contraception and management of pregnancy. Pediatr Med Chir. 2010;32(6):284-8.
13. Szekely P, Julian DG. Heart disease and pregnancy. Curr Probl Cardiol. 1979;4(6):1-74.
14. Faculty of sexual & reproductive healthcare, royal college of obstetricians & gynaecologists, faculty of sexual & reproductive healthcare Clinical guidance, contraceptive choices for women with cardiac disease, clinical effectiveness unit, JUNE 2014, ISSN 1755-103X.

CHAPTER 12

Multiple Choice Questions

1. **All of the following increases in pregnancy except:**
   a. Peripheral vascular resistance b. Heart rate
   c. Cardiac output d. Plasma volume

Ans. a. Peripheral vascular resistance

2. **Maximum increase in cardiac output occurs when:**
   a. First trimester b. Second trimester
   c. Third trimester d. Immediate postpartum

Ans. d. Immediate postpartum

3. **Which of the following is abnormal findings in pregnancy:**
   a. Lower limb edema b. S3
   c. Ejection systolic murmur d. Diastolic murmur

Ans. c. Ejection systolic murmur

4. **ECG changes normally seen in pregnancy except:**
   a. Shortened PR interval
   b. ST depression
   c. ST elevation
   d. Isoelectric low voltage T wave

Ans. b. ST depression

5. **The physiological basis for anemia pregnancy is:**
   a. There is a decrease in RBCs resulting in decreased oxygen carrying capacity.
   b. There is an increase in both RBCs and plasma with plasma increasing at greater proportion.
   c. There is an increase in plasma volume while RBCs count does not increase.
   d. There is an increase in plasma volume while RBCs count decreases.

Ans. c. There is an increase in plasma volume while RBCs count does not increase.

6. **Pregnancy is absolutely contraindicated in which of the following congenital conditions in which patient feels otherwise clinically well:**
   a. Cyanotic disease
   b. Fontan circulation

c. Eisenmenger syndrome
d. TGA with systemic right ventricle and mild dysfunction.

Ans. a. Cyanotic disease

7. **The appropriate time to start folic acid supplementation is:**
   a. Preconceptionally (3 months)
   b. Preconceptionally (1 month)
   c. As soon as the patient conceived
   d. Second trimester

Ans. b. Preconceptionally (1 month)

8. **Pregnancy is well tolerated in:**
   a. Stenotic lesions
   b. Regurgitant lesions
   c. Mixed lesion
   d. None of the above

Ans. c. Mixed lesion

9. **Most of the antiarrhythmic drugs belong to which category:**
   a. A
   b. B
   c. C
   d. X

Ans. a. A

10. **Most common arrhythmia seen in pregnancy:**
    a. Supraventricular tachycardia
    b. AV nodal re-entrant tachycardia
    c. Atrial fibrillation
    d. Atrial flutter

Ans. a. Supraventricular tachycardia

11. **Ventricular tachycardia is seen in association with which structural heart disease?**
    a. Hypertrophic cardiomyopathy
    b. Valvular heart disease
    c. Congenital heart disease
    d. Coarctation of aorta

Ans. b. Valvular heart disease

12. **Which drug is the drug of choice in long QT syndrome?**
    a. Digoxin
    b. Metoprolol
    c. Verapamil
    d. Flecainide

Ans. a. Digoxin

13. **When does peripartum cardiomyopathy generally occur (if it does)?**
    a. The last month of pregnancy to the first 5 months after delivery.
    b. The last 5 months of pregnancy to the first month after delivery.
    c. The last 5 months of pregnancy to the first 5 months after delivery.
    d. The last month of pregnancy to the first month after delivery.

Ans. a. The last month of pregnancy to the first 5 months after delivery.

14. What causes peripartum cardiomyopathy?

a. Unknown etiology
b. Sickle cell anemia
c. Atherosclerosis
d. Lung disease

Ans. a. Unknown etiology

15. In patients requiring cardiac transplantation, to bridge till transplantation what can be used?

a. Left ventricle assist device
b. Immunosuppressive therapy
c. Immunoglobulin
d. Anticoagulant

Ans. d. Anticoagulant

16. Echocardiographic findings suggestive of peripartum cardiomyopathy includes all except:

a. Left ventricular end-diastolic dimension >2.7 cm/m^2
b. M-mode fractional shortening <30%
c. Ejection fraction <0.45
d. Ejection fraction <0.60

Ans. b. M-mode fractional shortening <30%

17. At what time should an ANC with prosthetic valve switch to heparin during pregnancy?

a. 32 weeks
b. 36 weeks
c. 28 weeks
d. Postpartum

Ans. d. Postpartum

18. Chances of adverse outcomes in heart disease in pregnancy is increased during all of the following except:

a. At the time of labor
b. 4–5 days after delivery
c. 28–32 weeks of gestation
d. First trimester

Ans. d. First trimester

19. Pulmonary hypertension (PH) is defined as a rise in mean pulmonary artery pressure_____at rest as assessed by right heart catheterization.

a. 10 mm Hg
b. 15 mm Hg
c. 20 mm Hg
d. 25 mm Hg

Ans. c. 20 mm Hg

20. All of the following increases in pregnancy except:

a. O_2 consumption
b. Coagulability
c. Stroke volume
d. Cardiac output

Ans. c. Stroke volume

21. Riociguat is:

a. Endothelin receptor antagonist
b. Phosphodiesterase inhibitor
c. Guanylate cyclase stimulator
d. Prostaglandin analogues

Ans. c. Guanylate cyclase stimulator

22. Which of the following is false about anticoagulation in pregnant women with prosthetic heart valves disease?

a. Biosynthetic grafted-tissue heart valves do not need anticoagulation during pregnancy.
b. 3-hydroxy-3-methyl-glutaryl-coenzyme A reductase inhibitors (statins) are contraindicated in pregnancy.
c. Warfarin is associated with a risk of embryopathy between 12 and 16 weeks of gestation.
d. The risk of embryopathy seems to be low in women taking warfarin doses of 5 mg per day or less.

Ans. a. Biosynthetic grafted-tissue heart valves do not need anticoagulation during pregnancy.

23. According to risk assessment if total score ≥4 antenatally, consider thromboprophylaxis from:

a. First trimester
b. 28 weeks
c. 32 weeks
d. 24 weeks

Ans. b. 28 weeks

24. Insertion and withdrawal of a spinal catheter should be avoided within _____ of a subcutaneous dose of LMWH.

a. 6 hours
b. 12 hours
c. 24 hours
d. 48 hours

Ans. c. 24 hours

25. Which of the following crosses the placenta?

a. UFH
b. LMWH
c. Fondaparinux
d. Danaparoid

Ans. d. Danaparoid

26. All of the following requires monitoring of factor Xa level except:

a. LMWH
b. Fondaparinux
c. Apixaban
d. Dabigatran

Ans. d. Dabigatran

27. Which of the following is/are a contraindication to caesarean section under regional anesthesia?

a. Fontan circulation
b. Severe pulmonary hypertension
c. Severe aortic stenosis
d. Mechanical valve with full anticoagulation

Ans. a. Fontan circulation

28. Which of the following statements about the use of oxytocin in women with heart illness after a caesarean delivery is/are correct?

a. It results in a 50% reduction in SVR.
b. If at all possible, a bolus dose should be given.
c. If hypotension occurs, ephedrine is the vasopressor of choice.
d. In women with pulmonary hypertension, it should be used in conjunction with ergometrine.

Ans. a. It results in a 50% reduction in SVR.

29. Which of the following statements about contraception and pregnancy care in pregnant women with pulmonary hypertension is/are correct?

a. Oral contraceptive efficacy is reduced by endothelin receptor blockers.
b. Prostacyclin derivatives and phosphodiesterase inhibitors should be provided consistently to pregnant women with pulmonary arterial hypertension because they are the key contributors to a better prognosis.
c. When a woman with pulmonary hypertension becomes pregnant, termination is recommended and can be done safely.
d. The preferred technique of delivery is a caesarean section under general anesthetic.

Ans. a. Oral contraceptive efficacy is reduced by endothelin receptor blockers.

30. Tubectomy in a woman with heart disease is best done _____ after delivery.

a. 1 week
b. 2 weeks
c. Immediately
d. 48 hours

Ans. a. 1 week

Index

Page numbers followed by *b* refer to box *f* refer to figure, *fc* refer to flowchart and *t* refer to table.

T

U

V

W

X

Y